Parenting Different

How to raise your neurodivergent kids to be their authentic, awesome selves

SARAH HAYDEN

murdoch books

Sydney | London

Published in 2025 by Murdoch Books, an imprint of Allen & Unwin

Murdoch Books Australia
Cammeraygal Country
83 Alexander Street, Crows Nest NSW 2065
Phone: +61 (0)2 8425 0100
murdochbooks.com.au
info@murdochbooks.com.au

Murdoch Books UK
Ormond House, 26–27 Boswell Street, London WC1N 3JZ
Phone: +44 (0) 20 8785 5995
murdochbooks.co.uk
info@murdochbooks.co.uk

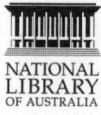

A catalogue record for this book is available from the National Library of Australia

A catalogue record for this book is available from the British Library

ISBN 978 1 76150 023 7

Cover design by Hazel Lam
Cover photograph from stocksy.com

Typeset by Midland Typesetters, Australia
Printed and bound by CPI (UK) Ltd, Croydon CR0 4YY

Murdoch Books acknowledges the Traditional Owners of the Country on which we live and work. We pay our respects to all Aboriginal and Torres Strait Islander Elders, past and present.

10 9 8 7 6 5 4 3 2

*To my beautiful family – thank you for sharing this
neurosparkly life with me. Without you I am nothing.*

*And to all the neurosparkly people I have the honour of
working with every day – thank you for trusting me on your
journey of courage, resilience, love and acceptance.*

Contents

Introduction

I don't know what led you to pick up this book today. Perhaps you are the parent of a newly diagnosed neurosparkly[1] child, or you are thinking of exploring a diagnosis for your child. Maybe you are a teacher or therapist working with neurosparkly people and simply want to learn more. Whatever your reason, congratulations on taking the first step to creating a better world, for wanting to find out more and how to better care for the neurodivergent kids in your life.

Thank you for investing in my book. It is truly an absolute honour to me that someone would use their precious time and money to read something I have poured my heart and soul into.

Parenting can be hard. Parenting our neurodivergent children can feel even harder. But it needn't be this way. Embracing neurodiversity means accepting, celebrating and

---

1 The dictionary defines 'neurosparkly' as a brain that has been dipped in colourful, sparkly glitter to make it much more awesome, also known as a neurodivergent brain. (This is absolutely not true, but it does prove how creative our neurosparkly brains can be.) There's nothing wrong with using the word neurodivergent, and you'll see it throughout these pages. But as you'll soon learn about me, I prefer to add a bit of extra sparkle wherever I can!

supporting our awesome, sparkly kids rather than expecting them to change. It means understanding that while they may do things *differently* to neurotypical kids, it doesn't make them *wrong* or in need of treatment. It means adjusting how we do things to help our kids manage everyday activities and tasks in ways that feel natural and normal to them. It means taking the pressure off our neurodivergent kids to behave in neurotypical ways, encouraging them to be themselves rather than hiding who they are by masking or changing their behaviours.

It also means taking the pressure off ourselves, as parents, to feel like we need to do things a certain way, usually due to a fear of judgement from *those* parents (you know the ones). All of this pressure is physically and mentally exhausting, for our kids and also for us. This book will help you discover new ways to parent differently, which may be just what you and your child need.

Who we are

Fifteen years ago, when my eldest daughter, Chloé, was first diagnosed autistic at the age of twelve, never in my wildest dreams could I have imagined I would one day be writing this book, as both a professional who works with neurodivergent kids, and as a proud parent of an incredible woman who is now known and recognised across the world – not in spite of her autism, but because of it.

Marie Claire's 2022 Rising Star of the Year; star of the worldwide smash-hit Emmy Award-winning Netflix series *Heartbreak High*, for which she won the 2022 AACTA Audience Choice Award for Best Actress and was a 2023 Logie nominee; *Vogue* cover girl; bestselling author; home owner . . . the list goes on and on and on – and I have a feeling she's only getting started. Not bad for a timid, selectively mute autistic girl who had no friends and absolutely hated school!

Little did I know on that diagnosis day, when I thought my whole world was falling apart, that I would one day be a part of the most incredible community with some of the smartest, most amazing, creative, quirky, unique and beautiful humans in the whole wide world. And that my daughter would be up the front, leading the change to radical acceptance, a hero and role model to other neurodivergent people around the world.

Fearless, brave, outspoken, loud, proud social-justice warrior and world changer – never would I have associated those words with that shy, terrified little twelve-year-old girl. And now they don't seem enough. What words can do justice to what Chloé has done so far? She is my inspiration. I want to be just like her when I grow up.

But before I properly begin, please allow me to introduce myself. My name is Sarah. I am a registered social worker and qualified equine-assisted psychotherapist, and I have worked primarily with autistic families for the past decade. I am also proudly neurodivergent, having been diagnosed with ADHD at the age of 48, after suspecting I was for many years. But, most importantly, I am mum to five of the most amazing humans on the planet: Chloé, 27, Gemma, 23, Hunter, 20, Wei, 16, and Fen, 12. I am also happily married to my best friend and lover of 30 years and counting, Ronnie.

With permission from Chloé and the rest of my family, I will be sharing the parts of her – our – story that have led to us to being here today and me writing this book.

I want this to be the book I wish I had been given early on in our journey. It is written from my perspective not only as a parent but also with the benefit of my professional experience with many neurodivergent people and their families. I am also blessed to have the wisdom of my incredible Chloé, who has carved out a life for herself I could never have imagined. She is doing everything – and more than – she ever dreamed.

Our family's journey has led me and my partner to discover ways of parenting that we were never taught growing up in a society that runs on systems designed for neurotypical brains.

From Chloé 🦋

Not all parents can become superhuman. I got lucky that my mum could. If you have not yet achieved that ability, I suggest you read this book. It might not teach you how to fly, but it will teach you how to be the warrior your child needs.

How to use this book

Day after day, I am contacted by parents, carers, teachers and therapists working with neurodivergent young people who want to know how they can better support them and provide a safer, more inclusive environment.

I have covered the topics people most commonly ask me about, from diagnosis to schooling, meltdowns, family life (including the big one, food), puberty and entering adulthood. You can read the chapters in order or jump straight to whichever topic appeals to you. There are also insights from Chloé and other neurodivergent people I'm lucky to know, and at the end of each chapter I have included a Q&A section that high-lights some of the most common questions that parents ask me. I hope you find this helpful and feel less alone knowing that so many are seeking the same answers as you.

> **IMPORTANT REMINDER**
>
> If reading any part of this book makes you feel like you *have* been doing it all wrong, or makes you feel like a shitty parent, just know we are all human and we've all been there. We all make mistakes, but it is never too late to learn and change.

My hope is that this book answers your burning questions and brings us one step closer to creating a world where everyone feels accepted and heard. I want to give us *all* permission to be our authentic, sparkly selves.

Settling in

Before you start actually reading this book, I would like to introduce you to a concept you possibly hear thrown about a fair bit but don't actually practise as much as you should (and yes, I am talking to myself here, too): this little thing called 'self-care'. An absolute must for *all* parents, even if most of the time it's a 'do as I say, not as I do' kind of thing!

Let me share a couple of common techniques I use with my own clients when they are feeling overwhelmed. They are great ones to teach your kids, too. You don't need any tools, and you can do them anywhere, even when you are driving, in a crowd or at work.

CALMING TECHNIQUES

- Five senses grounding technique: use your senses to identify five things you can see, four things you can touch, three things you can hear, two things you can smell and one thing you can taste. Doing this helps shift your focus, immediately grounding you, and calms the mind, alleviating anxiety in minutes.
- Five-five-five exercise: simply breathe in deeply for five seconds, hold your breath for five seconds, then breathe out for five seconds.

Right now, I just want you to take a big, deep breath and relax. Hopefully your little munchkins are in bed sound asleep (lol, one can only dream – we know our neurosparkly kids do not sleep!). Or, even better, you are lying on a sun lounge in the Bahamas with the warmth of the sun on your back and the sound of the waves crashing in the background (even bigger lol).

Wherever you are, grab a cuppa, a wine, or even a giant margarita – there will be absolutely no judgement from me; I would join you if I could – settle in, get comfy and read on.

If you are feeling anxious about this journey, I hope you can feel me here with you as you take each step. If I could reach out through the pages of this book and give you one of my famously big and tight mama-bear hugs, I would (only if you like hugs, that is).

Otherwise, just know that I get it. I have been where you are, and you've got this. You are the exact parent your child needs, and the reason I know that is because you have this book in your hands right now. You want to know how to do the best for your little bear cub, and that is enough.

Chapter 1

Parenting the neurosparkly way

I've written this book to help you support your child to unlock their full potential and, most importantly, live a happy life in which they feel loved and accepted. Together, we're going to embrace the fact that a diagnosis is not the end, but rather the beginning of a beautiful parenting journey. Let's start with a few basics.

What's with all these *neuro* words?

The word *neurodiversity* recognises and embraces the natural variations between all human brains and the ways they function. For much of the twentieth century, people whose brains worked differently from what was seen as 'normal' were institutionalised and often given horrific treatments in an effort to 'fix' them.

In the 1990s, autistic people, in particular, built an online movement to advocate for the idea that their different ways of seeing the world weren't 'wrong' or in need of a cure.

Neurodivergence, then, refers to these ways of being that have historically been treated as different from 'normal', or *neurotypical*. Neurodivergence is an umbrella term that includes the following ways of being:

- **ADHD,** or attention deficit hyperactivity disorder, shows up mostly as differences in the parts of the brain that we use to plan, focus on and carry out tasks.
- **Autism** describes differences in how a person socialises and communicates, thinks and processes information, moves and senses the world around them.
- **Bipolar disorder** can been seen as intense shifts in mood, energy levels and behaviour.
- **Down syndrome,** where a person is born with an extra chromosome, can result in distinctive physical features and differences with how a person walks, speaks, learns and plays.
- **Dyscalculia** looks like using atypical methods or having challenges in understanding number-based concepts.
- **Dyslexia** involves difficulties with decoding and composing written text.
- **Dyspraxia** refers to a brain's inability to plan muscle movements and carry them out.
- **OCD,** or obsessive compulsive disorder, may involve frequent unwanted thoughts that result in repetitive behaviours.
- **Tourette syndrome** is characterised by involuntary sounds and movements, or tics.

These neurodivergent identities also commonly occur together, due to the shared genetic, neurological and developmental pathways that underlie many of them. Some statistics suggest a more than 50 per cent co-occurrence of Tourette syndrome and

ADHD, while 50–70 per cent of autistic people also have ADHD. The problem is that due to the rigidity of single-diagnosis pathways (not to mention the enormous expense and time it takes to receive that single diagnosis), many people may not even be aware they have multiple neurodivergencies.

THE FOCUS OF THIS BOOK

While the neurodivergent umbrella is a broad one, in this book I focus on autism and ADHD, because I have the most personal and professional experience with those identities. I still think any parent on the journey towards discovering their child's neurodivergence will find the information in this book useful, but you can also find resources for other specific types of neurodivergence at the end of this book.

Different, not less

Because neurodivergent people are in the minority in our current world, this means that many of us will *mask* or camouflage our traits in an effort to fit into a society made for neurotypical brains. While neurotypical people may modify their behaviour to be more socially successful, the neurodivergent form of masking is mostly done to avoid negative consequences. This can cause extreme stress and lead to exhaustion, identity loss, anxiety and burnout.

I'm a huge believer in making your child's world as *neuro-affirming* as possible. This means you understand that every human in the world naturally has differences in their abilities and strengths. So rather than viewing neurodivergence as deficits or disorders, we understand and appreciate the unique talents and abilities of everyone without trying to fix them. In other words, we love and accept our kids just as they are.

Neuro-damaging (did I just make that term up? Hello, Urban Dictionary!) would be the opposite of neuro-affirming. This means thinking that neurodivergence is a problem that needs fixing. Or promoting the idea that neurotypical is the gold standard and trying to make our kids conform to whatever you think 'normal' is. (Even the word 'normal' sounds so bland and boooooring . . . neuro*sparkly* sounds so much more fun!)

Years ago, Chloé started using the phrase 'different, not less', and it has become our household mantra. Just because Chloé cannot read a clock or recite times tables, it does not mean she is *less*, she is just *different*. The things she is *amazing* at far outweigh the things she struggles with. Wouldn't you much prefer to be incredible at singing, or photography, or drawing, or know more about the giant squid or the black-eyed tree frog than you know about your seven times tables?

Now this part is really, *really* important – if you only take one thing away from this book, then this should be it. I want you to do everything in your power to encourage every neuro-divergent child you know (whether or not they have an official diagnosis) to be brave, be bold and be *proud*. They are what makes the world unique. They are what makes the world different and special and amazing. They are perfect just as they are. They don't need to change. They *are* the change.

A note on language

As awareness and acceptance of neurodivergence increase, the language around it is constantly evolving. I've done my best to use the terms and ideas that are broadly accepted at the time of writing.

While I have occasionally distinguished between some experiences of girls and boys, especially when it comes to the history of diagnosis and physical changes that occur during puberty, these mentions should be read to include anyone who has been assigned a particular gender at birth. Neurodivergent people are more likely than neurotypical people to identify as gender-diverse, so it's important that we allow everyone the space to find themselves under this umbrella.

When discussing neurodivergence, we must always aim to use language that is respectful, accurate and empowering. Instead of using terms like 'suffering from' or 'afflicted by', which imply negativity or pity, most people prefer identity-first language – such as 'autistic person' – which reflects pride in one's neurodivergent identity. This is why I use 'autism' rather than ASD, which, being short for 'autism spectrum disorder', keeps the focus on neurodivergence as a problem. Sadly, we don't yet have a term for ADHD that doesn't include the 'D' for disorder, but I'm sure we'll get there.

It's also crucial to avoid the outdated or stigmatising terms 'high functioning' or 'low functioning', which oversimplify the nuanced experiences of neurodivergent individuals. Instead, focus on describing specific strengths and support needs. By choosing words thoughtfully, we can foster an inclusive and positive world for our kids to grow up in. It is equally important to understand that the needs and abilities of neurodivergent kids can vary greatly from one day to the next. A child might appear to be 'high functioning' one day – where they are managing social interactions, schoolwork and daily tasks with ease – while the next day they may struggle significantly and appear to be 'low functioning'. This variability is completely normal and depends on a multitude of factors such as sensory sensitivities, emotional state, sleep quality or even changes in routine. Labelling a child as high or low functioning can be misleading as it doesn't capture the fluidity or full spectrum of their experience and abilities. Recognising this variability (which can change from one minute to the next) allows parents, and others in the child's community, to be more responsive and adaptable, providing the right support based on the child's needs at any given moment, without fixing them in place with labels.

Another word I've stopped using altogether is 'Asperger's' to refer to a specific type of autistic child, because it comes from Hans Asperger, believed to be complicit in the Nazi program that euthanised disabled children. So yeah, I don't want his name near my kids.

Of course, it's important to flag that the neurodivergent community is not a monolith, so some neurodivergent people may not agree with the views on language I've expressed above – and I will always support anyone's right to identify exactly how feels best for them.

Finally, I have changed the names of the gorgeous neurodivergent kids I work with whose stories I share in these pages, to protect their privacy.

How might neurodivergent traits show up?

Let's look at a few examples of how neurodivergent traits can be expressed. It's important to note at the outset that neurodivergent people all have unique presentations, so don't worry if your child doesn't fit neatly into the below descriptions – they are simply a rough starting point.

With autism, a growing number of researchers, including renowned autistic anthropologist and primatologist Dawn Prince-Hughes, argue that many (if not most) autistic people show certain human advantages, such as an unusual ability to pay attention to visual and auditory information, which may give them musical talents or a laser-like attention to detail. Autistic people are also often very direct with a strong moral compass. Neuropsychologist Isabelle Soulières says, 'It is true and scientifically proven that subgroups of autistic individuals have [certain] abilities that are better than non-autistic individuals.' Kate Cooper, a research fellow and clinical psychologist, adds that 'we now know that the *average* autistic person with even *average* characteristics of autism' – so not just the stereotypical *Rain Man*-like 'savants' – 'have strengths that set them apart from non-autistic people'.

Autistic people may struggle with socialising and maintaining eye contact, but their many incredible gifts can include:

- honesty, loyalty and reliability (such valuable traits for maintaining friendships and other relationships)
- absorbing and retaining facts (as anyone whose kid has a particular hyperfixation knows all too well)
- a methodical approach, making them fantastic at spotting patterns and analysing data (it's no surprise that many coders are autistic).

Some of the outstanding people who have either been diagnosed with or thought to have autism include Greta Thunberg, Albert Einstein, Isaac Newton, QuestLove, Darryl Hannah, Grace Tame, Steve Jobs, Hannah Gadsby, Michelangelo, Josh Thomas and Mozart.

While those with ADHD may have difficulty staying focused on tasks, their many strengths can include:

- hyperfocusing on one task for hours on end (what an *incredible* attribute for employees)
- being highly creative and able to see things from a different perspective
- having high levels of energy, which can be advantageous (except perhaps at 2 am).

Famous people with ADHD include Emma Watson, Justin Timberlake, Solange Knowles, Bill Gates, Clementine Ford and Jamie Oliver.

Superstars who are both autistic and have ADHD include Em Rusciano and our very own Chloé Hayden!

Dyslexic people are most commonly known to have trouble with reading and writing, but their advantages include:

- brilliant spatial reasoning (many dyslexic people excel in graphic design, engineering and architecture)
- incredible imaginations (many artists, actors and authors are dyslexic)
- exceptional problem-solving skills (many top entrepreneurs are dyslexic – including Richard Branson).

Other high-profile dyslexic people include Leonardo da Vinci, Jessica Watson, Danny Glover, Jackie French, Steven Spielberg, Jennifer Aniston, Mohammed Ali, Dick Smith and Anthony Hopkins.

An OCD person, such as singer Kelly Clarkson, may have brilliant organisational skills and attention to detail, while

Down syndrome people (such as model Ellie Goldstein) are often very strong in visual awareness and learning. Bipolar folk – let's hear it for the iconic Carrie Fisher – are usually highly creative and empathetic.

From Chloé 🦋

Something I admire about my mum and dad is that, even before I was diagnosed, they have always focused on my *cans* instead of my *can'ts*. My family is very strengths based. We speak a lot about the positives of our diagnoses and our disabilities. This is so massively important.

That said, we're not immune to the struggles of being disabled. We discuss those openly in our house, too. I see autism and ADHD as my superpowers, but I have my own kryptonite that comes along with them, and that's okay. That's part of human existence.

All of these strengths reinforce my strong belief that despite the stigma that has previously attached to those in the neuro-divergent club, we now know these people are simply *wired* differently, not *weird*, and we can start supporting them to be the best versions of themselves, whatever that may be.

So how can we parent our neurosparkly kids differently, wonderfully and more effectively? Let's start with a deep breath and a big-picture view.

Sarah and Belle's seven parenting don'ts

This list was written with Belle, an incredible young autistic woman I work with. Belle is absolutely slaying at life now but reports having a miserable childhood, due to her parents not understanding autism. With Belle's permission, I am sharing her heartbreakingly insightful reflections on how *not* to parent a neurodivergent child. These are the voices we need to listen to, and I am writing this book for amazing people like Belle and, of course, her parents, who I am sure did the best they could with the resources available at the time.

> ## REMINDER
>
> If reading this section makes you feel like you *have* been doing it all wrong with parenting your neurodivergent child, please be kind to yourself. Remember that no one has ever shown us how to do this. The journey is all about being open to growing and changing, so that we can support our kids in the way they need. When we know better, we do better.

1. Don't shit on your kid's special interests.

If your child is a Swiftie, do not try to make them love opera. Belle remembers becoming so excited and overwhelmed while watching a livestream concert of Taylor Swift, she started sobbing, shaking, screaming, flapping and yelling. Pure autistic joy! She had never been happier and could feel it right through her body . . . until her parents burst into her room, yelled at her for being ridiculous and immature, and told her to 'just stop'.

Wow. Way to burst a bubble and ruin a beautiful moment, Mum and Dad.

When Chloé was a young adult, her *obsession* with One Direction continued to gather steam long after every other teenager had grown out of it. She wanted all the merch, no matter how 'babyish' it was. The day One D announced their breakup, Chloé was utterly distraught. So that very day I drove around to every single Aldi supermarket, which had a big One D merch sale on, and I bought her all the pins, stationary, bedlinen and posters. I couldn't stand all the tacky merch in my home – it did not go with my decor whatsoever! But if One D were going to break Chloé's little heart by breaking up, the least I could do was buy her all of their merch.

Wait, that makes perfect sense, doesn't it? In a moment of what for her felt like genuine heartbreak, this was a small gesture I could make to show her I was listening and I cared. I didn't have to personally understand the devastation she felt, all I had to do was see *she* was feeling real pain and support her through it.

2. Don't hide your kid's diagnoses – or tell them to.

I am frequently asked by parents, 'When should I tell my child they are neurodivergent?' This just blows my mind. Secrecy around your child's diagnosis encourages a sense of shame. Kids will always pick up that something is going on, even if they don't know what it is. So when do you tell your child they're neurodivergent? As soon as you know. It can obviously be done in an age-appropriate way, and I will talk more about this in the next chapter. Just as we would never hide if our child had diabetes or wore glasses or had a hearing aid, we should never be ashamed of their neurodivergence.

Similarly, telling your child they won't be hired in a job or have friends or get a boyfriend if they reveal their neurodivergence can be so damaging. As Belle says, 'I already hated myself as it was. To have my own dad tell me to hide a huge part of myself confirmed to me that I was right to hate myself and be ashamed of who I was.'

My mission in life is to encourage people to be loud and proud of their neurodivergence rather than ashamed or embarrassed. I truly see it as something to be celebrated. If a child's own parents can't be positive and encourage acceptance of who they are, what is that telling them to expect from the rest of the world? And if their friends or boyfriend or employer do reject them for disclosing their neurodivergence, then they were simply not worthy of your child's awesomeness in the first place.

3. Don't be negative about your kid's neurodivergence.

Belle remembers that her father would refer to her autism as a 'condition', as if she was infectious. He would tell her that she was disabled and would be so for the rest of her life, so should learn to 'deal with it'. Because of how her parents and family treated her, she didn't find her home to be a safe haven, which is essential for neurodivergent kids. Belle felt the early sting of discrimination when she saw her parents treating her differently from her neurotypical siblings.

4. Don't play the victim or be an 'autism mum'.

Autism mums (or 'moms' in the United States) – ugh – what a bad reputation they have. The online Urban Dictionary describes an 'autism mom' as: 'A mother of an autistic child. Often considers herself a superhero for raising an autistic child, victimizes herself, and expresses negativity or grief about her child's condition. Likely supports Autism Speaks and the puzzle piece (both offensive to autistic people). Autism moms always know what's best for their children.' An autism mum sees her child as 'trapped' by autism, and she builds her identity around becoming her kid's saviour.

Now let me start by saying that you may simply identify as an 'autism mum' in the way that you can be a 'soccer mum' or a 'dance mum' . . . you may be just trying to find your tribe. It's absolutely priceless to have parents you can spend time with, empowering and supporting each other, or even just someone to sit and have a glass of prosecco with by the fire. But autism is more than an extracurricular activity, and, sadly, autism mums are notorious for wallowing in self-pity, loudly declaring how hard they have it because they have autistic kids.

Belle remembers that her parents constantly brought up in arguments with her how hard *their* life was because she was autistic – as if she was doing it to annoy them. They mocked her unregulated emotions and even told her she was to blame for their marital problems.

Don't play the victim card. Don't blame your kids for their diagnosis or your struggles. Don't label yourself an autism mum (unless you yourself are autistic, then go right ahead!). Life can be hard enough for our kids, so the least we can do is take responsibility for our own challenges.

5. Don't trivialise your child's mental wellbeing.

Neurodivergent people are at high risk of struggling with mental wellbeing (more on this in chapter 6). Given this landscape, we must do all we can to radiate positivity and acceptance for our children, supporting them in the ways they need.

When Belle was struggling with an eating disorder, however, her parents blamed her for wasting their food and their money. 'They said I was a stupid and selfish little brat and just doing this for attention,' she recalls. There are many ways to deal with an eating disorder. This is not one of them. Most people are not starving themselves intentionally, and making it about you is not going to help anyone.

Please, if you suspect a loved one may have an eating disorder or is starting to get a dysfunctional relationship with food, seek professional advice and support immediately. The same goes for any other mental health concern your child may experience.

6. Don't misinform your kids about their neurodivergence.

Belle remembers that her parents often told her she had no empathy because she was autistic. It was only when she became an adult that she realised, like many autistic people, she actually felt things *more* deeply than neurotypical people. But her parents making her feel like she was a heartless monster had already done untold damage.

Telling your child they have no empathy is a sure sign you lack empathy yourself. What an awful thing to say to someone. Autistic people may not show empathy in the same way as others do, but it is a misconception that they do not demonstrate or show empathy. In fact, some research suggests many autistic people may feel the emotions of others – especially their negative ones – more intensely than neurotypical people do. I know this is certainly true in our house. Chloé has always felt things so much more deeply than others and for others, particularly for animals. When you watch an autistic girl rescue the snails in the rain so no one stands on them, or chew up food in their mouth to spit into the mouth of the baby bird they just rescued, you begin to understand the very definition of pure empathy.

7. Don't be ignorant. Educate yourself!

One of the most important things we can do as parents – and humans – is to educate ourselves on things that matter and are relevant to those we love. If our child is diagnosed as neuro-divergent, we owe it to them, and ourselves, to understand the potential challenges they may face. We know that quite a number of neurodivergent people struggle with executive dysfunction, meaning that they may have difficulties with managing time, completing tasks, planning, organising and prioritising.

Belle remembers that her parents had no understanding of her challenges and called her lazy whenever she couldn't do something. She grew up thinking there was something wrong with her until she was old enough to learn about the relation-ship between her autism and executive dysfunction. 'If I could learn about it,' she said, 'surely they could, too.' You don't have to have all the answers, but being willing to join your child on this journey is so important and will have such a positive impact on your relationship with them.

Sarah's seven parenting dos

Here are my top tips on how we can parent like a pro to help our neurosparkly children thrive.

1. Love what they love (or at least fake an interest in it).

Showing you are interested in your child's current hyperfixation is a sure-fire way to connect with them. If your child loves nothing more than dressing up as Spider-Man and heading to Comic Con, then get your Batman suit out ready for an awesome weekend experienced through the eyes of your child. I guarantee you will be their instant superhero. And, hey, your child's obsession with One Direction may even lead to your very own special interest (did I mention I was in the top 0.01 per cent of Spotify Top Fans for Harry Styles in 2024?).

One of the girls I work with, Andie, is the biggest Swiftie I've ever met. I mean, every Swiftie is very passionate, but this girl is *next level*. Her mum told me Andie's new stepfather was having trouble connecting with her, as he was not only new to parenting but also new to autism and the obsessive special interests that can accompany it. Andie wanted to attend the Taylor Swift concert more than anything in the world . . . (like *anything*) but she had missed out on tickets and Mum couldn't stand going to concerts due to her own sensory sensitivities. So we hatched a plan – her stepfather became a diehard Swiftie, listening to her music every time he was in the car with his stepdaughter and even sharing facts he had been learning about her. Andie was sceptical at first, but when her stepfather surprised her with tickets to Swift's concert in another city, she was convinced. I still laugh at the thought of him enduring an eight-hour road trip wearing sparkles, friendship bracelets and listening to Taylor on repeat . . . my actual definition of a nightmare, and probably his, too (sorry, Swifties, but I will take Harry over Tay Tay any day of the week!). But his willingness to jump on board with Andie's special interest has done wonders for their relationship.

It's also good to remember that it is often your child's special interests that help them connect with peers. All of Chloé's friends have come from her special-interest groups. And, in fact, her career began because she was blogging about her special-interest groups, so you never know where these brilliant obsessions may lead.

2. Accept your child, quirks and all.

Our biggest job as parents is to accept and validate our child's unique personality, however it's expressed. We can often have unrealistic expectations of our children, and when they don't meet these, it can lead to stress, anxiety, disappointment and even anger on both sides. Instead of fighting against their quirks, we need to learn to love, encourage and accept them. After all, 'normal' is just a setting on a washing machine.

One set of parents I worked with were a bit concerned about their daughter, Norah, whose fascinating quirk was her intense passion for the weather. She would spend hours watching weather forecasts, memorising cloud types and tracking storm patterns across different regions. Norah would excitedly point out a cumulus or nimbostratus cloud while I nodded along, agreeing that they did look like different pretty bits of cotton wool.

Initially her parents were worried their daughter's fixation might limit her social interactions or academic growth, and that she was missing out on 'normal' childhood experiences, including friendships with others who weren't quite so 'focused'. However, after learning more about the importance of embracing neurodivergent interests, Norah's parents decided to shift their perspective. Instead of constantly trying to divert her attention to other 'more normal or acceptable' activities, we discussed what it would mean to encourage her special interests. They began buying Norah books on meteorology, setting up a weather station in the backyard and encouraging her to learn all she could. They excitedly searched weather maps together and scrolled social media pages of other nephophiles (see, there are so many others just like her that they have a name!). By accepting and supporting their daughter's unique interest, Norah's parents not only helped her thrive academically but also, more importantly, found new ways to connect with her, ensuring she felt loved and accepted. I am sure Norah will be a very cool meteorologist one day!

3. Create a safe home where their needs are met, and they know they are loved and supported.

The world can be big and scary for kids, especially neurodivergent ones, and home is the one place where everyone should feel safe, loved and supported. By ensuring your child has the freedom to be themselves and their own space to do so, we can encourage them to remove their masks and recharge their batteries. I always say, 'You're only neurodivergent when you step outside your home.' This might look like setting up a quiet sensory-friendly corner in the house where they can retreat when feeling overwhelmed, or it could mean allowing them time alone in their room to decompress after a long day. Giving your child this space isn't about isolating them, it's about acknowledging their need for solitude to recharge and self-regulate. By providing these safe, private areas, you're showing your child that their needs are valid, and that it's okay to take a break when they need one.

4. Prioritise your kid's comfort and wellbeing over the opinions of others.

Opinions are like arseholes – everyone has one. At some stage you have to get to the point of not caring what others think of you or your children. Remember, what other people think is none of your business. If your child needs to sit in church wrapped in a weighted blanket with their ear defenders on, then that's what you encourage them to do. If Mrs Busybody tut-tuts about their awful manners, you kindly tell her to mind her own business. As long as your child is not disrupting the service or causing harm to others, let them be and ask others to do the same.

One of the families I work with is Indian, and they place a huge importance on food in their weekly family gatherings, including everyone, young and old, eating extremely spicy curries. Unfortunately, their son, Nishant, prefers nuggets and chips to rogan josh and beef vindaloo, much to his grand-parents' horror. The grandparents saw this as a rejection of their culture. I discussed with Nishant's parents how this was more than just a preference, and that he had a strong sensory aversion to spicy foods that quite literally made him sick. I explained that they needed to listen to their son's needs and help their family understand that he was on a special diet and needed to eat these foods (it's not entirely a lie, the special diet for autism *is* often nuggets and chips!) and to just take those foods for him when they attended shared family meals.

5. Put their mental health above everything else – *every single thing.*

Pay attention to this one: it saves lives. The *only* thing that matters when it comes to our kids is maintaining their mental (and physical) health. The most important thing you can do is actively listen to your child, validate their feelings and create an environment where they feel safe expressing themselves.

Establish consistent routines and provide predictability to help reduce anxiety and build a sense of security. Encourage and support their unique interests and needs, even if it means deviating from societal norms or expectations. Be prepared to advocate for their mental health needs with schools and other institutions, ensuring that the right accommodations and support systems are in place.

One of the teenage girls I work with, Olive, hated Monday mornings at school so much she would make herself physically sick all Sunday in anticipation. She had reached the stage where she couldn't sleep on Sunday nights. Every other day was fine . . . it was just Monday mornings. I was able to discover from talking to Olive that she absolutely hated the all-school assembly, which was only held first thing Monday – the noise of 500 kids crammed into the tiny school hall, the bright lights, the squeaking feedback from the microphones, the smells of the gym toilets right next to where she was allocated to sit . . . it was a sensory nightmare that was clearly having an enormous impact on her mental health. Was it worth it? *Absolutely* not! Was the solution so easy it was a no-brainer? *Absolutely* yes! As soon as we made the decision that Olive's Mondays would now start at 10 am – straight after school assembly – the Sunday night sickies disappeared.

6. Understand their particular sensory sensitivities and executive dysfunction.

Your child will teach you everything you need to know about them. It is up to you to listen and learn. If your child tells you their school tights feel like stinging nettles, validate this, even if they feel like velvet to you. This can be difficult to accept if your child absolutely hates hugs and you love them, but you have to understand it is not personal. Allowing them to give or deny consent to physical touch with you is also amazing practice for handling trickier social situations as they grow up.

One of my incredible clients, Meg, is the most creative little girl who absolutely hates hugs – in fact, all touch is strictly out of bounds. She has sweetly found alternative ways to express her affection to the rest of her family (who are, ironically, all very big huggers). Meg absolutely loves carefully crafting handmade cards with beautiful words and pictures, which she presents with great pride and often for no reason at all. These personalised expressions of affection allow her to connect with her family in a way that is comfortable and meaningful for her – without a hug in sight. I had to wipe away a little tear when I was presented with an exquisite home-made card during one of my sessions with her. It felt *just* as good as a hug – or maybe even better, since I knew how much thought had gone into it.

7. Stand your ground with 'experts'.

In this era of online parenting books, family bloggers and endless therapeutic professionals, it can be easy for parents to feel overwhelmed by 'experts', but I am here to remind you that *no one* knows your child like you do, no matter how many fancy bits of paper hang in their office. Listen to your gut and your intuition, and learn to trust yourself, while continuing to learn everything you can about your child. If you do decide to seek guidance, it doesn't remove or diminish your authority as a parent or caregiver – it actually reinforces and enhances it.

You've got this!

If you worry after reading this chapter that you may not have got it all right so far, or you are worrying about the mistakes you may have made along the way, please remember that most of us parents are just muddling our way along pretending to know what we are doing, attempting to adult and looking for an *adultier adult* because we don't feel very adult ourselves. (Or is that just me?!)

Our kids deserve to know and understand their brains and their bodies, their needs, their strengths and their struggles. And everyone needs someone in their corner to celebrate, support and advocate for them. An amazing adult (or, even better, a whole tribe of amazing adults) who doesn't give up, who will fight for them and commit to learning all they can, even if it means unlearning or relearning what they thought they knew, or going against the grain. Sometimes that means doing things differently, because sometimes different is amazing and beautiful and exactly what you – and your kids – need.

Q: MY CHILD HAS JUST RECEIVED A DIAGNOSIS. IS IT WRONG THAT I'M SCARED FOR THEIR FUTURE?

A: It is completely natural to feel scared when your child receives a new diagnosis, and I would be lying if I said I didn't feel a little bit the same. It's a big moment that can bring up so many concerns for their future, especially when you don't know much about it or have heard horror stories. Remember, a diagnosis is not a limit or an end, it is a starting point for understanding your child's unique strengths and challenges.

It is also helpful to think of it not as something 'new', but simply a name for how your child has always been. Every single child is capable of achieving great things, and with the right support, they can thrive in ways that are meaningful to them. Embrace this diagnosis – or discovery – as a tool that can help you advocate for and tailor support to your child's individual needs. Focus on their abilities, celebrate their progress and remember that many neurodivergent people go on to live incredibly fulfilling and successful lives.

You are not alone on this journey – in fact, you have just joined the most awesome, supportive, beautiful community of people you could ever hope to meet. Congratulations! And *welcome*. I just know you're going to love it here.

Q: I FEEL SO MUCH GUILT AND SHAME ABOUT HOW I HAVE PARENTED MY NEURODIVERGENT CHILD SO FAR. I DIDN'T UNDERSTAND THEIR NEEDS, AND I FEEL LIKE I'VE FAILED THEM. HOW CAN I MOVE FORWARD?

A: First of all, it's important to acknowledge that you're not alone in feeling this way. Many parents of neurodivergent children experience guilt or regret about past actions, especially when they learn more about their child's unique needs. Actually, let's face it, I think every parent feels guilt at some point. What's important now is the commitment you're showing to grow, learn and do better.

Parenting is a journey, and we don't always have a clear map. You were doing the best you could with the knowledge and resources you had at the time. Recognising that you could have approached things differently is a sign of growth, not failure. It's never too late to build a more understanding and supportive relationship with your child. Every step you take towards understanding them better is a step in the right direction. You are doing the hard and courageous work of learning, adapting and loving them for who they are.

Chapter 2

Diagnosis (aka discovery!)

Many of you will be at different places in the journey towards a diagnosis (or, as I like to call it, 'discovery') for your child. Perhaps you are wondering whether to pursue a diagnosis but aren't sure where to start. Or maybe you have already received their diagnosis, and looking back, you wonder how on earth you missed it.

It is understandable to be feeling a range of emotions at this point: fear and uncertainty about what is to come, or possibly shame and guilt for not recognising it earlier. If it makes you feel any better, my 23-year-old daughter Gemma was diagnosed with both ADHD and autism at the age of 22, and I am supposed to be the expert!

Neurodivergence can present so differently from one person to the next. In so many ways, my two girls couldn't have been more different in their presentation, and yet – just as it had with Chloé – it made so much sense. Gemma had already received a dyslexia diagnosis several years earlier, and during an ADHD assessment her psychologist suggested that she also be screened for autism, which came back as a big neurosparkly *yes*!

Wherever you find yourself, I hope this chapter can bring you to a place of acceptance and then joy about the discovery that comes with a diagnosis.

Our first story of discovery

Looking back, I can see all the signs – now that I know what they are, of course. Hindsight is a wonderful thing. From when Chloé was incredibly young, we always referred to her as 'quirky'. Being young, inexperienced parents, and this being our first child, we had no one to compare her with. From the moment Chloé was born, she was a difficult sleeper. It felt like she never slept. Like, ever. If she did, it was in tiny bursts, a few minutes here and a few minutes there – and only if she were being held tightly or rocked. She was colicky, uncomfortable and whingy, and leaving her alone in a bassinet or cot simply was not an option. She was, at all times, attached to one of us.

As she grew older, she complained about the intensely itchy woollen tights that she wore, and we would joke that she was like the princess in the classic story *The Princess and the Pea*, in that she could feel anything and everything – no matter how small or seemingly insignificant. Even the smallest of tags on her clothing caused her so much pain and discomfort, it was like she was wearing a cactus. I became the master of removing them. If I left even a single stitch there would be screaming and tears, and not just from her!

From the age of around eighteen months when she took her first steps, Chloé walked on tippy toes or with her feet on a strange angle, wearing one side of her shoes out before the other (something she still does). She adored music and dancing but would fall over constantly. She despised loud noises and lights despite being very, very noisy herself.

As a primary schooler, Chloé would sit and recite facts she had learned from various encyclopedias she had read late into the night, then kindly offer these facts to anyone she came across. Curiously, she appeared neither concerned nor interested in whether the people she was sharing with were *actually* listening – it seemed more important to her to just put the information in front of as many people as possible that there were, in fact, 60 species of kangaroos.

She was gifted at drawing and writing stories, but her handwriting was completely illegible (she would explain that her hands couldn't keep up with her brain). At school, she was uninterested in the other kids and preferred to spend free time collecting insects and saving injured birds. Most teachers seemed to love her, her classmates not so much. (The teachers who *didn't* love her, meanwhile, were the ones she would correct all the time. She was right, they were wrong, and funnily enough, they did not like that one little bit!)

It was at high school that we – and Chloé herself – really noticed how different she was. She seemed so young and naive compared to the other girls. Her school reports were rapidly getting worse and consistently described her as disorganised, messy, loud and chaotic. One day I received a phone call from a concerned library teacher asking me if I was aware that Chloé hid in the library during every single recess and lunch break, and quietly ate her food in the toilets to avoid others. Every day ended in tears as she was subjected to the torment of bullies who preyed on her differences. Life was getting more and more difficult – for her and for us.

When one of her teachers quietly pulled me aside and asked if I had ever considered taking Chloé to see an educational psychologist, I was genuinely shocked and confused. I had never even considered doing such a thing. After all, our child was wonderfully perfect just as she was. But I was also at a loss for what to do about the emotional distress she was experiencing. So not long after, I found myself sitting in a room with my daughter and an educational psychologist.

Our initial appointment lasted a couple of hours and included the psychologist taking a full history of Chloé's childhood, as well as all the information that had been given to her from the school. At the end, the psychologist casually looked over her glasses and said to me, 'There are a lot more assessments to be done, but at this stage I believe your daughter has Asperger's.' (Please see my rant on page 12 about why we don't use 'Asperger's' these days. We're always learning and growing and doing better!)

Seeing the look of utter confusion on my face, the psychologist handed me an encyclopedia-sized book, *The Complete Guide to Asperger's Syndrome* by Tony Attwood, and told me to start reading it, and to come back in a fortnight.

I'm so ashamed to admit this now, but as I walked out to the car – the big fat book under one arm and my subdued, confused daughter following behind me – I started crying. Really, really sobbing. Years of parenting my precious, quirky and at times fragile child flashed before me, and my heart broke.

As soon as I sat in the car, I picked up my phone and googled *Asperger's syndrome*. There, in black and white, was the exact description of my daughter.

Chloé then picked up the book and quickly read the blurb. 'Mum, this sounds *exactly* like me!'

As I found myself crying even harder, I nodded in agreement with her.

'Is it really that bad?' she tearfully asked.

Seeing the concerned look on her face, I realised I had to put on a brave front. 'No, of course not, it's nothing,' I said.

'If it's *nothing* then why are you crying so much?' she asked.

Touché.

I would like to add here – contrary to what Chloé believed at the time – that I was not crying over the fear of having an autistic child as much as I was for the overwhelming regret and sadness that I had not known about it for thirteen years. I would also like to add, in hindsight, there is actually not much I would have done differently if I had known. We (very) successfully – in my humble opinion – parented Chloé exactly as she needed (*most* of the time, no one's perfect) and instinctively made adjustments as we went along. It's one of the reasons I so strongly believe that parents are the best professionals when it comes to their own kids' needs.

The following months were an emotional whirlwind of very expensive and lengthy appointments and assessments until we finally got the official diagnosis (discovery), some 58 pages long. Chloé Hayden: AUTISTIC.

My first-born child. My perfect daughter. My gorgeous, smart, quirky little genius. Autistic?! But she was *nothing* like *Rain Man*! And, sadly, in the year 2010 that was the only autistic representation in the media. Not that there is anything wrong with *Rain Man*, but Dustin Hoffman's character sure as heck didn't look like my little girl, so you can understand why autism was not something I had considered. (Thank God for Quinni on *Heartbreak High*! Rocking autistic representation since 2023.)

I was absolutely shocked, confused, devastated but also there was a tiny part of me that was relieved that we finally had an answer to why Chloé had been struggling so much, especially at school.

I found myself reading whatever I could get my hands on and was astounded to see that pretty much every description of autism in females summed up my daughter perfectly. How could we have missed it? How could my family have missed it? We were well educated, my dad was a doctor, my mum a nurse, and not one of us had realised there was something going on with my daughter.

None of it made sense, and yet suddenly everything made perfect sense.

The older Chloé got, the more 'autistic' she appeared to become. Even when we began to school her from home, she needed me to help her with each and every step of her schoolwork, and I began to see firsthand why school had been so hard for her. On the flip side, so much of her anxiety and sadness seemed to disappear overnight.

Chloé was always intelligent, an incredible writer with very mature insight, yet she struggled to cross the road or read a clock. At that time I thought she would never go on to further education, never hold down a full-time job, and I prepared for the possibility that she might live with us forever, which I was on board with. As long as she was happy and mentally okay, I was okay. I could not see her ever having a partner and could not even dream of her becoming a mum. But we continued to encourage her, celebrating her unique qualities and accepting her limitations, as we saw them.

My attitude has changed enormously since she was first diagnosed. I am no longer scared. I'm informed and I'm her biggest advocate. She is unique, she is beautiful and she is creative. We love her and we love her autism. I know when she

From Chloé 🦋

Reading this story of my diagnosis, I am reminded of how little I knew then, including that I thought I had 'ass burgers' or something to do with asparagus. On the other hand, being diagnosed just confirmed what I already knew about myself.

I knew from as young as four that I wasn't like the kids around me. I would hold Mum's hand tighter when people my age walked past me, already painfully aware of a neurotype I didn't have. Similar to how those others knew that I was different, I did, too.

Society has this idea that humans have to be a certain way. But the world doesn't work unless there's difference. Neurodivergent kids are people who pioneer what *different* can mean. Yes, there are struggles but look at what we can do. Our brains are magic. If society focuses only on the struggles, they'll never see the beauty of it all.

I get messages every day from parents saying that their kid has been diagnosed but they're scared of telling them because they don't want their child to have a label. The fact is, your kid already has a label. My labels in school were 'stupid', 'disorganised', 'loser'. I got called all those horrible words. When I got my diagnosis, my label became 'autism'. I chose that label myself. Now instead of thinking I'm 'lazy', I understand how my brain works and have systems in place to help me.

I would love to think that one day saying you're autistic will be just like saying you're left-handed. Oh, by the way, I *am* left-handed!

needs hugs, and I know when she needs to be left alone. I also know how wrong I was to project my fears and limitations onto her – that was not my role as a parent.

I am also absolutely positive the psychologist knew within *seconds* of meeting Chloé that she was autistic, and we probably could have saved ourselves many months and many thousands of dollars for the autism assessment. In our very first session with her, the psychologist walked out and formally introduced herself, holding out her hand to shake Chloé's. Chloé responded by pointing out that the poster of whales in the waiting room was wrong, as it contained factually inaccurate information, so she should *not* have it hanging up. The psychologist looked at me with a knowing smile as Chloé barged past her and into the room to line up the toys in her clinic.

I now know that smile. It's the exact smile I give to my own clients' parents all the time.

Your diagnosis journey

Given my experience, I often notice that someone has autism within five minutes of meeting them (except for my own husband or second-eldest daughter). My daughter tells me it's my 'tism radar! But day after day I come across families who have tried for years without luck to seek answers for their kids, and even parents in their forties and beyond, who only finally got a diagnosis themselves after their child did. I am so thrilled that they are finally understanding who they are and how best to love, support and understand themselves.

Getting a diagnosis can not only help you understand your child's needs and how best to help them, but also bring a great sense of relief – for both you and your child. If they have always felt 'different' or have never fitted in, this may help to explain things. Diagnosis can create opportunities to connect with others and feel connected through shared interests.

Diagnosis can also bring with it financial and practical support. It is easier to receive support in the school, university or workplace with an official diagnosis, and most countries (including Australia) have legislation in place that requires institutions to make reasonable adjustments for those who are diagnosed.

It can be a long and expensive journey to receive a diagnosis, and at times you might feel it is not worth following through with it. But getting the additional support can make such a difference to you and your child.

Just because you have an official diagnosis, of course, doesn't mean you have to actually use it. However, having it in your back pocket gives you the ability to use it if needed.

Self-diagnosis is also perfectly acceptable in the neurosparkly community. And hey, who wouldn't want to belong to this super cool group of people?

Now when people come to me telling me their child has had a recent diagnosis (discovery) of neurodivergence, I tell them 'Congratulations!' and I mean it. With the right support, our kids can be the most incredible people who truly light up this world. Some of the most amazing, inspirational, colourful and life-changing people in the world are neurodivergent. What a boring world it would be without them!

Where to start

You know your child better than anyone, so research the most appropriate place to get a diagnosis. In Australia, a diagnosis can be completed by a single qualified professional such as a psychologist or psychiatrist, or by a multidisciplinary team. It can be done through the public health system (likely a long wait and a low cost) or the private system (a short wait and a high cost). Regardless of where you are, a good starting point is your local GP.

Go in with all the reasons you are seeking the diagnosis, including signs and symptoms you have recognised (more on this below). There is nothing wrong with reading checklists – there are plenty available on the internet – and you could even print them out and write beside them the corresponding signs you see. Not every person is going to tick every box, though, and that is fine, too.

If you are seeking a diagnosis for a child who displays the less classic, more overlooked traits of neurodivergence, which can frequently happen with girls and gender-diverse kids, as well as some boys, find a team that specialises in your child's gender identity. Time and time again I have witnessed the girls I support 'failing' (or should I say 'passing'?) their autism assessment at mainstream public diagnostic services, when I was able to tell *immediately* that they were autistic. When the families have then opted to pay for a private assessment with a team specialising in female diagnoses, they were quickly diagnosed as autistic. Do not ever be afraid to get a second opinion, not just when seeking an assessment or diagnosis but in *any* medical care for your child – or yourself, for that matter. While this private pathway is unfortunately not cheap, it may be well worth it to get the diagnosis, which can then lead to the support and understanding they (or you) need and deserve.

For kids diagnosed with ADHD, taking medication may be an option to deal with some of the challenges that they face.

There are a number of different medications, and it's often a matter of trial and error to see if the benefits outweigh the side effects. In Australia, only a psychiatrist can prescribe this medication, and they won't accept a psychologist's assessment of ADHD, so keep this in mind when weighing up which diagnosis pathway to walk down.

It's useful to be aware of the sorts of behaviours and feelings to look out for when considering whether to seek a diagnosis for your child. I've covered the main ones for autism and ADHD below, but you'll find resources to start the journey for other possible diagnoses at the end of this book.

Diagnosing autism

Almost everything we know about autism comes from studying boys, which means almost every checklist used to diagnose autism is still based on symptoms found in boys. While boys are still more likely to be diagnosed than girls, recent research suggests that this may be due to girls' traits being treated differently due to gendered social norms. Add to this the fact that autistic children are less likely to identify with the sex they were assigned at birth (perhaps identifying as transgender, non-binary or gender-queer), as well as the fact that racial bias can make a diagnosis more difficult for people of colour, and it's clear that we need to be looking out for a wide range of characteristics when it comes to autistic presentations.

Many autistic girls, and even some boys, particularly those without an intellectual disability, are more likely to be creative and clever at hiding their symptoms, which is known as masking. They are like chameleons, changing to fit in with their environment. In school, teachers will be naturally less inclined to notice the kids who are not displaying disruptive behaviours. This can make it much harder to diagnose autism, resulting in a missed diagnosis, a *mis*diagnosis, or a much later diagnosis and therefore missed opportunities for support. Girls and women are commonly misdiagnosed with things such as bipolar, borderline personality disorder, anxiety and depression.

Here are some of the areas where kids may show characteristics of autism, with a range of examples to show you the different ways in which these traits may show up.

Social interaction

Many autistic children avoid eye contact as they find it uncomfortable or don't place the same importance on eye contact as neurotypical people do. They also might not respond to their name, which could either be related to hearing, speech or language delays, or, again, because they do not value social responses in the same way that neurotypical people do.

Autistic kids may correct people or misinterpret what others are saying. Others can read our kids as being nasty, but it is more likely to be that they have difficulty reading social cues and body language. Many autistic people also struggle with impulse control, which can mean they are more likely to interrupt conversations and have trouble taking turns.

In my equine therapy rooms, I have a play area with lots of toy horses and stables. Just about every one of my neurosparkly clients will arrange the horses in precise rows by colour and breed. They are perfectly happy in their own world engrossed in the soothing activity of sorting. Parallel play is a common behaviour of many autistic children, who may prefer to play *alongside* their peers or siblings than directly *with* them. It's a valuable reminder for parents that social engagement looks different for each child, and every form of play has its own worth.

Differences in social interaction can often be overlooked in girls, as they will often identify someone they want to be like – a popular girl at school, an actress on their favourite television show or a character in the novel they are reading – and then intently study and mimic them. This comes at great emotional cost, however, as suppressing their authenticity can ultimately lead to burnout and depression.

There's one area of social interaction that Chloé has never suppressed, though: she says exactly what she thinks and does not understand why anyone would lie. This trait can cause problems with peers – and the general public. As a young child, she walked up to a woman and told her she was 'very, very fat'. While this lady was indeed on the larger side, she was entirely unimpressed by skinny little Chloé informing her of this. I copped an enormous amount of abuse from this rather angry lady. And as we were walking quickly back to the car, Chloé turned back around to her and loudly proclaimed, 'But you are very, *very* fat.' The entire car ride home was spent with me attempting to educate Chloé on thoughts that are best kept inside our head.

Special interests

Autistic special interests can be recognised by their level of intensity. While many kids will love animals, autistic kids will love them with a passion, knowledge and understanding not seen in their neurotypical counterparts.

As a child, Chloé would want to sleep in her horses' stables and would sit under a tree to read to them. Even when she was very young, Chloé knew more than anyone about animals and could recite more facts than most encyclopedias, zookeepers or museum guides. She could tell you about different species, the correct scientific names and breeding cycles of animals you had never even heard of. I remember one time we were at Sea World listening to the presenter talking about dolphins when Chloé raised her hand to correct them. It turned out seven-year-old Chloé was right, and the marine biologist was wrong.

While special interests in boys may sometimes be the obvious one of trains (*Thomas the Tank Engine* on repeat, anyone?), in girls they can be overlooked because they may align with behaviour that is seen as socially acceptable for girls, such as an intense love of reading.

Repetitive movements or noises

Often known as 'stimming', these can be a way to communicate, a way to deal with overwhelming sensations and movements, or simply an activity that feels good. Common stims include hand flapping, rocking, jiggling, spinning, pacing, snapping fingers or biting fingernails.

Repeating words or noises (known as echolalia) is another stim seen frequently in children. One of my young clients, Theo, repeats everything his mum says when they come to see me. So when we're going out to see the horses, his mum will say, 'It's time to put on your boots and coat.' Without missing a beat, he will respond with, 'It's time to put on your boots and coat,' in the exact same tone and rhythm as his mum. For Theo this echolalia is a natural part of how he processes language. Sometimes it's his way of showing that he has heard and understood what's been said, even if he doesn't respond with his own words.

More subtle stims that may be overlooked include watching the same TV program over and over, re-reading the same book or writing about the same topic or event.

Emotional regulation

Many autistic children find it challenging to understand and regulate their emotions. They might suppress their emotions publicly but have massive meltdowns at home. I call this the 'Coke bottle' effect. Our kids are being shaken all day long, and when they walk in the door of their home where they feel safe, the lid explodes and the Coke fizzes everywhere. I have been in many care-team meetings at school when the teachers have implied that maybe the problem is at home, because they do not see the behaviours the parents are describing. No, that is because often meltdowns are reserved for the special and safe people in their lives. So if your child is saving them just for you, be thankful they have a safe place to fall.

Aggression can be an autistic child's way of trying to communicate when their needs are not being understood. When a young autistic client of mine, Toby, who is completely nonverbal, suddenly started biting his carers repeatedly, it caused a lot of concern (and pain) among his team. People were getting hurt, and this new behaviour was frustrating and upsetting for everyone, but no one could identify why it had suddenly started. One day I had a light-bulb moment. Why do babies dribble and bite hard? When they are teething and their teeth are hurting them. So I suggested Toby go to the dentist, and sure enough, he had a tooth abscess that required immediate treatment. Of course, Toby was unable to *tell* us, so he was *showing* us. Sometimes we need to listen with more than our ears.

Strong sensory sensitivities

This may look like an aversion to particular sounds, smells and textures. For example, clothing tags that feel like cactus, and woollen tights that feel like stinging nettles. Lights that are so bright and hum so loudly that they cause migraines. Walking down the laundry aisle of the supermarket can be almost impossible with so many strong unnatural chemical smells competing for our attention.

Even when Chloé was a baby, she would scream if I put uncomfortable clothes on her until I took them off. Being my first child, and a girl, I loved to buy her beautiful outfits from my then-favourite store Pumpkin Patch. The dresses were frequently made from taffetas, wools and nylon, and while she looked exquisite, they were clearly not comfortable. Chloé would scream relentlessly until I took them off and replaced them with a $4 Kmart fleecy tracksuit, which she was happy to wear 24/7, much to my horror and embarrassment.

Some autistic children may dislike being touched, hugged or held, due to it feeling uncomfortable or even painful. This does not mean your child doesn't like affection, they may just show it in other ways. Other autistic children love being touched, hugged or held, and if they are sensory seeking, they may love deep-pressure hugs.

Sensory sensitivities may show up as a fussiness with food – wanting to eat only white foods or foods with certain textures, not wanting food to touch or being overly sensitive to types of foods, for example: 'All red foods make me feel sick.'

Love of routines and predictability

Many autistic kids like to know what to expect during the day and do not cope well with unexpected changes. Chloé, for example, has always liked to know what we are having for dinner. She explains that with so many uncertainties and variables during the day, it makes her feel safe and less stressed at least knowing how the day will end. So I keep a whiteboard on the fridge where I write the meals for the week.

Likewise, when a substitute teacher suddenly appears in class because our kid's regular teacher is unexpectedly off sick, this can cause great stress for them. Ensuring we are notified about changes like this can mean the difference between a good and a bad day. For *everyone*.

Motor skills

Autistic kids may walk on tiptoes or have an unusual gait. They may be uncoordinated and clumsy, having difficulty with seemingly simple tasks such as tying shoelaces, catching a ball and balancing. Their handwriting may be illegible and exhausting to produce due to fine motor difficulties.

Competitive team sports are often highly anxiety producing for our neurosparkly kids, and they will frequently be the last chosen for teams due to lack of friends and sporting ability.

Sleep

There are many reasons autistic children have problems sleeping, including difficulties with relaxing and winding down. This can look like not needing much sleep, taking a long time to get to sleep, being nocturnal, needing to co-sleep, or sleeping tightly swaddled or with weight on top of them.

Even when Chloé was a newborn, she required constant touch and weight on her to sleep. As a toddler, we would frequently fall asleep next to her cot with one of our hands lying on her tummy. You would think she was sound asleep and commando crawl backwards out of her room, only to be startled with a loud 'tummmyyyyyyy', which was her demanding you come back and rest your hand heavily on her tummy again.

In order to get some peace and quiet, some nights we would fill gloves up with sand and leave them on her tummy so she would think it was us. (She was far smarter than we were, though, and quickly picked up on our game. She was entirely unimpressed!)

Following scripts

This may look like bossing 'friends' around and scripting and directing their play, but it can also mean a love of following literal scripts: autistic children are frequently exceptionally talented in the arts, music and drama. I was always amazed watching Chloé as a young girl, selectively mute and painfully shy, but put her on a stage and she would shine with confidence. She explains this is because she did not have to come up with the words herself or face the unpredictability of not knowing what someone else would say, as everyone was following the script.

Collecting and ordering objects

Our kids may develop extreme attachments to inanimate objects, which become very real to them. Chloé once fell in love with an old stuffed deer as we passed the window of an op shop. It was love at first sight for the filthiest, smelliest, most germ-ridden toy I had ever seen. She started crying as soon as she saw it and for another half an hour on the way home. She got so hysterical about *saving* the deer that I had to turn around and go back. She couldn't bear to think of it alone in the shop without someone to love it. She loved that deer like it was real – after it had been washed a thousand times with Dettol in the washing machine. (Ironically, Chloé has a general aversion to dirt and germs, apparently unless they're found on a smelly deer from an op shop.)

Autistic children will often *collect* toys – this can be anything, from shells to erasers, cars, pencils or crystals – but not actually *play* with them. One girl I worked with had a huge Barbie collection, just like her friends. However, unlike her friends, she didn't play with them but preferred to line them up or categorise them according to something like their hairstyles.

Don't forget, autistic traits are not as clear-cut as these lists. As the saying goes, 'when you meet one person with autism, you have met one person with autism'. If you suspect your child might be autistic but their traits don't fit neatly into the boxes above, it's worth making a list of the reasons behind your thinking and doing more research or speaking to a healthcare professional or others in the autistic community to see if anyone else's experiences resonate with those of your child.

Diagnosing ADHD

As with autism, the classic understanding of how kids present with ADHD has narrowly focused on boys who seem like they've drunk too much red cordial and are spinning on their heads in the middle of the classroom. While, of course, some children with ADHD do act like this, ADHD can also present more as inattentiveness, or a combination of inattentiveness and hyperactivity. These traits, particularly in girls, kids who are gender-diverse and kids from marginalised backgrounds, may look quite different from the stereotypical hyperactive white boy, which puts them at risk of being dismissed or misdiagnosed. So it's important to do your research and be aware of the range of ways in which ADHD can show up.

Hyperfocus

While the full name for ADHD refers to an attention 'deficit', this can actually be quite misleading. Kids with ADHD can frequently become hyperfocused on a particular activity, losing track of time or ignoring other (usually more boring) tasks. That's a problem that often comes up in the classroom, where a child with ADHD may struggle to put their paintbrush down when the bell rings to signal the end of art class, because they haven't yet finished their sunrise. Or, at home, they might play video games so intensely that they forget to eat, sleep or even go to the toilet. In some kids, this may be characterised as disobedience, but it really stems from an inability to easily swap between tasks.

Time blindness

Time blindness is a common challenge for kids with ADHD, making it hard for them to sense the passage of time. Jason is a twelve-year-old boy with ADHD. Every morning his parents struggle to get him ready for school on time. Despite setting alarms and reminders, Jason often loses track of time. His mum will remind him to get dressed, but when she comes into his bedroom half an hour later, she finds him sitting on his bed with one sock on, deeply absorbed in the book he found under his pillow from last night. Even when his parents tell him, 'We are leaving in fifteen minutes,' it simply doesn't register like it might with another child.

To Jason, fifteen minutes feels the same as 30 minutes or five minutes – they are all completely abstract. Jason cannot break down the time needed to do something. He simply cannot process that he has fifteen minutes to eat breakfast, brush his teeth, pack his bag, get his shoes on and hop in the car. Unlike his mum, he genuinely doesn't feel the urgency until the very last minute, when Mum is screaming and the morning has turned chaotic.

By the time they rush out the door, Mum is angry and Jason is upset and confused.

Sensory sensitivities

While sensory sensitivities are more commonly associated with autistic kids, many ADHDers also struggle with sensitivities to input such as loud sounds or bright lights, which will often distract them from the task at hand. So a kid with ADHD may get distracted from doing their work at school because they can hear the lights buzzing, or the wall clock ticking, or because the kid next to them is making noise – and they usually won't be able to refocus on their work until that sensory stimulus stops or is otherwise managed.

Decision overload

Decision overload is another common problem for children with ADHD. Where there is an abundance of options, it is difficult for them to process and evaluate each one. Their brain works overtime to weigh up the pros and cons for every decision, but rather than narrowing down the choices, they become frozen by the sheer number of decisions. This leads to emotional overload, and in the end they feel so stuck, they are unable to make any decisions at all.

Sally is a ten-year-old girl with ADHD. When her parents took her to the toy shop to spend her birthday money, Sally was excited to choose a gift but quickly became overwhelmed. There were so many choices – games, soft toys, craft, stuffed animals – the list was endless. Her parents tried to help by making suggestions, but this only made her more anxious, as she was so worried about choosing the wrong gift and now she felt added pressure to make a decision quickly. After an hour in the store, Sally was feeling so overwhelmed by not being able to choose that she started to cry.

Impulsivity

The hyperactive part of ADHD may often show up as a child interrupting or talking over the top of others. While this may mean our kids are labelled as rude, it can actually come about in a few different ways. They may be emotionally dysregulated and have difficulty controlling their reactions, or they may feel the need to respond immediately so that they don't forget what they wanted to say. This impulsivity can even come from excitement: so many beautiful neurosparkly kids love to connect with others around their interests and may burst into conversations simply because they want to get involved and contribute to what's going on.

Losing things

One of the very real downsides of having a child with ADHD is how often you have to replace an essential item they've lost. This is linked to challenges in maintaining organisational focus. Back when Chloé was still going to school, she would catch the bus, following a long bushy path from the bus stop to our property. She'd often walk in the door barefoot, feet filthy after trekking through the muddy swamp along the way. I'd ask, 'Where are your shoes?' and she'd say, 'I lost them.' When I pressed her to remember if she'd had her shoes on the bus, she'd think for a bit and then say, 'I think I left them at school.' So she'd made it onto the bus and the whole walk home without even noticing that she was no longer wearing her shoes! On the day we finally pulled her out of school (more on this in chapter 5), the lost property collection was full to the brim with Chloé's stuff. It basically looked like her bedroom.

SOME KEY INDICATORS OF NEURODIVERGENCE IN KIDS

- sensory sensitivities
- repetitive behaviours and routines
- special interests
- anxiety or aggression
- social or communication difficulties
- troubles with sleeping

Q: SHOULD I TELL MY CHILD THEY ARE NEURODIVERGENT? IF SO, WHEN?

A: Should you tell your child they are neurodivergent? Absolutely! Exactly at what age is up to you, but in my opinion the day *you* find out is when *they* find out. Many people are concerned a 'label' may make someone feel broken; however, most newly diagnosed adults have found the exact opposite to be true.

Giving your child a name for their differences is their right and gives them a better understanding of themselves. It is highly likely your child already feels different to others, so in many cases they are hugely relieved to hear these differences have a name – and a community of kids who are similar.

I believe these conversations can become a natural part of general discussions around how everyone is unique and has their own strengths and weaknesses. Observations can be as simple as 'Daddy has to wear glasses to read and Mummy doesn't', or 'Grandma has to wear a hearing aid to listen but Grandpa doesn't', 'Aunty is wonderful at maths but your uncle is much better at English', or 'Your sister is left-handed, but your brother is right-handed like you'.

It is so important to normalise the fact that we all have things we are good at and enjoy, and all have things we struggle with and don't like doing. You can explain in simple terms that everybody's brains – just like their bodies and other features – are different. Most children need very minimal simple information that can be built on the older they get. You may decide to get a professional to help with explaining the diagnosis to the child, or you may use the help of books or YouTube tutorials. A simple conversation may start with, 'Do you remember we went and saw Janine (the psychologist), and she asked you lots of questions and played games with you? Well, Janine thinks you might be autistic.' It can be while watching autistic figures on TV such as Julia on *Sesame Street*. 'Do you see how Julia needs to have quiet times just like you sometimes? Well, that's because Julia is autistic – just like you!'

If you choose to hide your child's diagnosis from them, you may inadvertently teach them it is something negative to be hidden and ashamed of. Positive neurodivergent identity needs to start in the family home – ensure *you* are ready by identifying where you are up to with your own feelings about the diagnosis, as you do not want to become distressed or emotional while having this discussion. The longer you keep it secret, the bigger a deal it will seem, and this delay may end up causing far more problems than it solves.

Q: HOW DO I TELL OTHER PEOPLE MY CHILD HAS BEEN DIAGNOSED AS NEURODIVERGENT?

A: While your child absolutely has a right to know they are neurodivergent, sharing their diagnosis with the rest of the world is a little different. There is no shame in being neurodivergent, but they have a right to privacy, too. I believe the best way to decide who needs to know is to think about this: if there is a situation in which someone will be working closely with your child in an ongoing capacity, and your child may require some accommodation, modification, support or understanding from them, then those people should know. Some examples of these people may include: teachers, babysitters, therapists or sports coaches.

If your child is at school, sharing the formal diagnosis with those teachers working directly with them is crucial in ensuring they get the support and understanding they need. The school cannot make appropriate and reasonable adjustments without the evidence of the diagnosis.

If you have close family and friends who can be a positive support to both of you, then you may also choose to share this information. Some people choose to send an email with factual information in it; for example, how the diagnosis may impact your child, and the behaviours your family and friends are likely to see and how best to respond.

There may be situations in which you partially explain adjustments a child may need without fully disclosing a diagnosis. For example, a child may attend a three-day summer soccer camp, which is only a temporary relationship, so you may choose to simply give the coach enough information to support your child without disclosing the full diagnosis: 'Piper may need reminding to take her jumper off when it gets hot, as she doesn't always feel the heat in the way others do.'

Then there are people who do *not* need to know your child is neurodivergent. The lady serving you in the grocery store, your child's peers in their class, and even some family and friends. I have worked with some parents who have actively chosen not to tell their own families about their child's diagnosis, as they have already known the response will be negative and unhelpful. One beautiful mother of one of my clients told me she had to keep both her child's *and* her own recent diagnosis secret from her own mother, the child's grandmother, because she 'didn't believe in autism' and was very negative about it. It was so heartbreaking to hear the child explain that they had to hide their autism diagnosis from their own grandmother, but it was the best plan for their own mental health. Sadly, some people's friendship circles and even family dynamics may change after a diagnosis, depending on people's support and reactions, but ultimately it's about keeping your child – and you – safe.

Q: WHAT IF MY CHILD DOESN'T RECEIVE A DIAGNOSIS WHEN I THINK THEY ARE NEURODIVERGENT?

A: There is certainly the possibility your child is, in fact, *not* neurodivergent. There are other things that can be mistaken for it, including developmental, speech or hearing delays and even trauma. However, in my experience, if a parent is adamant their child is neurodivergent – and in this day and age, most parents are well informed and well educated about it, having done a lot of reading and research before seeking a diagnosis – then it is more likely they are than not.

If you strongly feel a therapist has misdiagnosed or missed a diagnosis, do not be afraid to explain to them why you think this is so and perhaps point out where in the diagnostic report they have incorrectly represented your child. Remember, you have likely been with your child 24/7 for many years, while the therapist may have spent a few hours with them, at most. If you feel they aren't listening, or you cannot provide this feedback, you can always seek a second opinion. Take the report and your concerns to the new professionals with your own feedback, including concise points on what you believe they have missed. You are the expert on your own child. You are also the best advocate for your child, and this may be the start of your journey of learning how to amplify their voice – so embrace it!

Q: WHY IS MY CHILD SUDDENLY MORE NEURODIVERGENT AFTER THEIR DIAGNOSIS?

A: I have had many parents ask me this. Recently diagnosed teens and adults will often ask the same about themselves or say a friend, partner or family member has commented this to them after they reveal their diagnosis.

Some people who ask this seem almost accusatory, as if they believe the recently diagnosed person is now changing their behaviour just to fit their new diagnosis.

I think there could be several reasons for this. The first is that often when an neurodivergent person understands and accepts their diagnosis, they realise what they may have seen as character flaws are just part of being neurodivergent. They may start to accept rather than repress these neurodivergent parts of themselves – they may finally feel allowed to let the mask drop and be their full selves.

Another, less positive reason that a person may seem 'more neurodivergent' is that they may hit a breaking point where they are not actually able to mask anymore. This is usually linked to what is known as neurodivergent 'burnout', which I'll cover in more detail in the next chapter.

Chapter 3

Neurosparkly nervous systems

Parenting . . . no one gives you a road map, so most of us are just winging it and hoping for the best. It wasn't until I was an adult (and I am talking 50 years old) that I realised none of us knows what we are doing. We're all just big kids trying to raise little kids, really.

Parenting a neurodivergent child is an extraordinary journey filled with unique challenges and profound rewards. Each day brings a deeper understanding of the diverse ways in which our children perceive and interact with the world. Throw in a fragile neurodivergent nervous system, and it's no wonder we sometimes feel like we're going to have our own little nervy b (which sounds *so* much cuter than a nervous breakdown, don't you think? Another one to add to the Urban Dictionary, perhaps!).

Ronnie and I had Chloé when we were both at the tender age of 23. The minute she came into our lives, we were absolutely besotted. She was the most exquisite baby and we couldn't have been more in love. Instinctively, we adjusted our routines entirely to fit her needs. If she needed to be rocked the whole time she slept, we did it. If she needed to sleep in our bed every night, she did. If we had to drive the car for hours at a time to get her to sleep, then off we went. As long as she was in our arms 24/7, she was a pretty happy baby. What we know now is that the repetitive and rhythmic motion of rocking and gentle movement can calm a baby's nervous system, helping them feel more grounded and connected. Thankfully I didn't have to go back to work, so for the first five years of life Chloé was attached to my hip and this suited me – and her – just perfectly. It got us through until it was time for school, which is when the issues really started (see chapter 4).

Many neurodivergent people have nervous systems that are more sensitive to sensory input than a neurotypical person's, making nervous system dysregulation a common challenge. This simply means it's easier for your child's nervous system to be overloaded and tip over into a meltdown or shutdown. It's important to understand that meltdowns and shutdowns are *not* just big temper tantrums, which means they require an entirely different response. While I don't want to turn this into too much of a science lesson (*not* my favourite subject at school) it can be useful to know a bit about what's happening inside your child's body so you can start to figure out how best to support them.

Nervous system info dump

The nervous system is the body's communication network, and it has two main parts. The brain and spinal cord are the central nervous system, which controls everything we do, from breathing to walking, thinking and feeling, playing a crucial role in regulating our bodily functions, from our heart rate and blood pressure to digestion and our emotional responses.

The nerves and other sensors make up the peripheral nervous system, which sends information to the brain and spinal cord about what needs doing, then carries the commands that the brain issues in response back around your body. Within this peripheral system sits the somatic nervous system, which looks after voluntary actions such as moving your arms or legs, as well as the autonomic nervous system, which takes care of those actions our body does automatically, such as breathing, sweating or shivering.

The autonomic nervous system has two modes: the parasympathetic state, which initiates rest and digestion; and the sympathetic state, which initiates our danger response. When our brain senses a threat, the sympathetic nervous system will prime the body physically to respond in one of the following ways, depending on the type of threat, how our brain is wired and our previous experience:

- Fight or flight: these are the classic ways we humans have responded to danger since the earliest days of dealing with predators such as tigers (or people who are mean to our kids). Our sympathetic nervous system releases adrenalin, which makes our heart beat faster and readies our muscles for action, giving us the energy boost we need to either fight the danger or run away from it.
- Freeze: if our brain decides that fighting or fleeing isn't an option, it may prime us to 'freeze', or play dead. This usually involves bringing the parasympathetic nervous system on board to decrease our heart rate and make our body stiff or numb, in the hope that the danger will pass us by.

These nervous system responses are critical to keep us alive in emergency situations, but we're not able to sustain them over long periods. The problem is that prolonged exposure to stress – which is everywhere in our hectic modern world – can lead to these responses being triggered by non-threatening situations. This can keep our body in a permanent state of fight, flight or freeze, which can have very damaging results.

Neurodivergent sensitivities

As I discussed in chapter 2, neurodivergent people often have a range of sensory sensitivities, all of which can overload their nervous systems, triggering those danger responses and contributing to an increase in meltdowns and shutdowns. It might be helpful to think of a meltdown as the fight-or-flight type response and a shutdown as the freeze type response.

The neurodivergent brain operates like an internet browser with 100 tabs open at once. Every time my tech-head son walks past my computer, he says to me, 'Mum, you'll drain your battery so fast with all those tabs open,' as he points to the 37 tabs lining the top of my computer screen, while rolling his eyes at my obvious incompetence.

My response is always the same: 'Haha, you think *that's* bad, you should see the number of tabs open in my brain.' I laugh . . . and then I cry, because constantly having soooo many tabs open in my mind is utterly draining and exhausting. Sometimes I cannot close them, no matter how hard I try. Because our neurodivergent brains – like an overloaded computer – are trying to process an overwhelming amount of information taken in from an overstimulating world, they often drain quickly, regularly running completely flat, and they also take longer to recharge.

Anxiety is also common in neurodivergent people. The nervous system has to work so much harder just to 'fit in' with the neurotypical world, and is often on high alert, which can leave the body feeling stressed.

Calming your child's nervous system is crucial for maintaining overall wellbeing. The good news is there are a number of fairly simple and effective techniques you can use, including:

- Deep breathing: engaging in slow, deep breathing exercises activates the parasympathetic nervous system and reduces stress. The Cosmic Kids website has a great range of fun breathing exercises to engage kids in this practice.
- Mindfulness and meditation: these practices promote relaxation and help manage stress responses. Try the soundwalks on ABC Kids Listen for a beautiful break.
- Physical activity: regular exercise helps reduce tension and improve your child's mood.
- Sensory activities: using weighted blankets, listening to calming music or engaging in gentle touch like massage can help bring a sense of calm.
- Nature play: spending time in nature has been linked to lowering levels of the stress hormone cortisol and boosting mood.
- Sleep: getting enough sleep is crucial for nervous system recovery and stress management. Right now you're probably laughing or rolling your eyes at the thought of your child getting better sleep, and I *so* get that. A few things that *may* help your child wind down for bed include warm baths, gentle music and their favourite bedtime stories (depending on their age). Some people swear by melatonin or a warm glass of milk and a snack. If all else

fails, you can do what we had to do, and that's letting them go to bed watching their favourite movie on repeat. It was honestly the *only* thing that worked. They got sleep, we got sleep – so don't judge!

- Nutrition: consuming a balanced diet and proper hydration supports the nervous system. Again, a nutritious diet and neurodivergent kids don't always go hand in hand, but we do our best. Just remember, every child is unique, so experiment to find what works best. A good dietician or nutritionist may be able to help.
- Structured routines: maintaining a consistent daily routine provides a sense of stability that may reduce anxiety.
- Professional support: counselling and therapy (see chapter 6) can provide strategies and support for managing stress and anxiety.
- Hobbies and interests: giving your child opportunities to pursue these can provide an enjoyable and fulfilling distraction and a sense of achievement.

By regularly practising these calming activities with our kids, we can reduce their stress, improve their mood and increase their capacity to focus and cope with daily challenges. This balance is essential for both their physical and mental health, which in turn can minimise the frequency and impact of meltdowns and shutdowns.

Stimming

Quite simply, stimming, or self-stimulatory behaviour, is the use of repetitive movements or sounds. For neurodivergent people, stimming can be a natural way to release built-up energy and regain a sense of calm. Interestingly, in some trauma therapies people are now essentially being taught to stim. EMDR (Eye Movement Desensitisation and Reprocessing) and somatic experiencing use rhythmic or repetitive movements that are similar to stimming to help people process trauma and soothe an overactive nervous system. These therapies recognise the value of self-soothing behaviours, showing that what might look like fidgeting to some is actually a valuable tool for emotional regulation. Embracing stimming as a therapeutic practice highlights the importance of allowing children to engage in the movements or sounds they need to feel safe and centred, proving once again that the best support often comes from respecting their natural instincts. So you could say stimming is a primal form of self-regulation – once again proof that neurodivergent people are superior beings!

Everyone, neurodivergent and neurotypical alike, stims at times. Clicking your pen, biting your nails, playing with your hair or tapping your feet are all examples of stimming that most people do every day, often without even realising it. And because most people stim in these ways, they're quite socially acceptable.

Some examples of stimming behaviours that are associated more with neurodivergent people – and which can be less socially acceptable – include hand flapping, rocking back and forth, finger flicking, or repeating words or phrases (sometimes known as echolalia).

Stimming can be helpful for emotional regulation, a way to 'cope' when your nervous system feels overstimulated. It can help to bring a sense of calm within the body when the environment feels anything but. These behaviours can provide comfort, reduce anxiety and help with focusing. They can also be expressions of pure joy, done because they feel good!

One of the teenagers who comes to see me, Phoebe, struggles with self-harm, depression and suicidal thoughts. She comes to me straight after school – a place where she is bullied relentlessly for being different – so when her car pulls into the driveway, you can see the sadness, pain and suffering on her face. The moment Phoebe hops out of the car and spots the ponies trotting over to meet her, her whole face beams with joy. Without thinking, she begins to flap her hands and spin in circles, her laughter echoing throughout the paddock. The ponies all come to witness and join her in this joy, playfully cantering in circles around her. To Phoebe, this isn't just movement, it's her way of expressing pure, unfiltered happiness. Stimming is her body's natural response to an overwhelming rush of joy – like a dance that's been perfectly choreographed to her emotions. For her, stimming isn't just about regulation, it's a beautiful celebration of feeling truly alive.

Stimming can be helpful in different ways depending on the type of neurodivergence: someone with ADHD may stim to help them focus, whereas an autistic person may stim to calm themselves when lights or sounds are overwhelming.

Unless stimming is harmful to the person doing it or the people around them, there is no reason at all to stop it. Instead, the stimming child may simply require acceptance or adjustment from the people around them.

However, if a child's stimming does become harmful – such as head banging, skin picking or pulling out hair (known as trichotillomania) – it's essential to find safer alternatives that meet the same sensory needs. Approach the situation with understanding and compassion. First, observe what triggers the harmful behaviour – stress, frustration, boredom? Once you understand the cause, offer substitute activities that provide similar sensory feedback, such as squeezing a stress ball, plucking feathers or fur from a toy, or squeezing 'pimples' from a gel pimple-popper ball. (Yes, this is *actually* a thing. They are the most gross and beautifully satisfying silicone toy, with lots of gritty little bits of pus that you can squeeze out. They are disgusting but also heavenly!) Remember, the goal isn't to eliminate stimming but to ensure it's safe and supportive. Encourage your child to communicate their needs and preferences, reinforcing the idea that they have control over their self-soothing behaviours. With patience and creativity, you can help them find healthier ways to self-regulate, keeping their nervous system happy without the risk of injury.

STIMMING TOOLS

Stimming tools can be a game changer for neurosparkly kids (and adults), providing a safe and effective way to manage sensory needs and emotions. These tools come in various forms, designed to offer tactile, visual or auditory stimulation that can help self-soothe or focus. The key is finding the right tool that matches your child's unique preferences and sensory needs, turning stimming into a positive and supportive part of their daily routine.

While you certainly do not need to buy all of these, it can be useful to have a few on hand for your child. Leave them in the car, scattered around the house (in dishes or bowls if you can't handle the clutter) or in their school bag, if the school allows it – if not, you may have to speak to the school about making accommodations.

Commonly used stimming tools include:

>>>

- Fidget toys: these small handheld gadgets that spin around a central bearing are perfect for keeping fingers busy and providing repetitive motion. Whether they spin or have buttons to press, these provide tactile and kinesthetic stimulation, helping your child find calm and focus.
- Squeezy (stress) balls: soft balls that can be squeezed to relieve stress and stimulate the hands.
- Slinkies and tangle toys: twisting and turning toys that provide a satisfying tactile experience.
- Chew toys: silicone necklaces, bracelets or pendants designed for safe chewing offer oral sensory input for kids who enjoy mouthing objects.
- Sensory brushes: these can be brushed on the skin or hair to provide calming tactile input.
- Weighted blankets: heavy blankets that apply deep pressure help to calm the nervous system and provide a sense of security.
- Sensory bottles: clear bottles filled with water, glitter and other objects, which swirl around when shaken, offering visual stimulation and a calming effect (these are so fun and easy to make, too).
- Textured fabrics: swatches of different materials such as velvet, corduroy or fur, which provide varied tactile experiences and are ideal for children who find comfort in touching different textures.
- Rain sticks: cylindrical instruments filled with small pebbles or beads that create soothing sounds when tilted, providing auditory stimulation – again, such easy ones to make.
- Liquid-motion bubblers: small, clear containers filled with coloured liquids that bubble and flow when flipped, offering visual intrigue and a calming focus.

- Putty: a malleable substance that can be stretched, twisted and squeezed to exercise the hands and fingers. The easiest putty recipe in the world is simply a cheap hair conditioner mixed with cornstarch and some food colouring.

Meltdowns

I am sure almost every single parent of a neurodivergent child has been accused of their child having a *tantrum* when it is actually a *meltdown*. In fact, you may have even accused your child of this yourself – I know I certainly have been guilty of making this mistake. It's hard to deal with those judgey looks and scathing comments when your child is lying in aisle three, screaming and thrashing arms and legs around, causing the most epic scene.

But while tantrums and meltdowns may look similar, there is actually a very big difference between them. A tantrum is usually only seen in younger children intending to get a particular response, so it is most often goal-oriented, intentionally manipulative behaviour. On the other hand, a meltdown is an intense response that can happen at any age, and is usually due to sensory overload or overwhelming situations beyond the person's control, with no purpose, goal or manipulation behind it. While a child (including a neurodivergent one) may have a tantrum about the fact that you wouldn't buy them a toy or a chocolate bar while at the supermarket, a meltdown is more likely to be triggered by the supermarket's fluorescent lights or overpowering smells, leading to sensory overload. Meltdowns are our sympathetic nervous systems triggering a fight-or-flight response to a perceived threat.

Meltdowns require understanding, not judgement. I will never forget years ago after Chloé had just finished an epic meltdown, in a moment of my own frustration I thoughtlessly said to her, 'Wow, that was *so* hard for me.' She looked up at me, tears streaming down her face, and said, 'If you think that was hard for you, think about how hard that was for me.' Out of the mouths of babes.

Meltdowns can be different for autistic and ADHD children, although there may be some overlap in how they manifest.

For autistic children, meltdowns are often triggered by sensory overload, changes in routine or overwhelming emotions. During a meltdown an autistic child might become very agitated, crying, yelling or even injuring themselves. This is their nervous system's response to feeling overwhelmed or unable to cope with the current environment.

For ADHD children, meltdowns might stem from frustration, emotional dysregulation or an inability to manage impulses. These meltdowns can resemble tantrums, because of their intensity and the way they seem to come from a place of frustration or defiance. However, it's important to recognise that these reactions are often beyond a child's control.

In both cases, it's critical to remember that meltdowns are not intentional behaviours but rather involuntary responses to being overwhelmed. Understanding these differences and the underlying causes can help you provide support tailored to the individual needs of your neurodivergent child.

Triggers

Meltdowns can be triggered by a number of factors. Common ones include:

- sensory overload, or overstimulation, coming from intense sensory input such as loud noises, bright lights, strong smells, crowded places or excessive amounts of activity
- unexpected changes in routine or disruptions to daily schedules
- emotional stress, such as frustration arising from confusing social interactions
- communication difficulties, such as being unable to express needs or feelings
- sensory sensitivities, including physical discomfort from clothing tags, textures or temperature changes
- unmet needs, whether hunger, thirst or fatigue.

Understanding the particular triggers for your own child is important in creating supportive strategies that may help to prevent or manage meltdowns.

From Chloé

An autistic person's level of functioning changes minute to minute, day to day, based on where they live, how burned out they are, their gender, their race, their living situation and many other factors.

Recognising the triggers or early signs of a meltdown helps. I know when I exert myself with a big day of acting or doing a conference speech that the next few days are going to be hard. My loved ones and I know a meltdown is coming, so we plan ahead for it, which saves me so much energy. The preparation doesn't stop the meltdown, but it allows me to experience it as safely as possible.

Early warning signs

Once your child has been triggered, they will usually show signs that a meltdown is imminent. While everyone is different, early signs can include:

- increased agitation, including signs of frustration, irritability or restlessness
- reacting more strongly to sensory inputs like loud noises, bright lights and crowded spaces, such as your child covering their eyes or ears
- difficulty regulating emotions, including more rapid mood swings, heightened or disproportionate emotional responses, or intense reactions to minor triggers
- physical symptoms including pacing, fidgeting, clenching fists and an increased heart rate (a sports watch that monitors your child's pulse can be helpful to determine this)
- verbal outbursts, including shouting, crying or noises of distress
- not being able to concentrate or appearing overwhelmed.

Recognising the early signs can give you time to take proactive steps to manage the situation and hopefully reduce the severity and length of the meltdown. Minimising a meltdown starts with proactive strategies that help manage triggers before they escalate. Establishing a predictable routine can provide a sense of security, reducing anxiety and the likelihood of sudden outbursts. Sensory breaks are also crucial; create a calm, quiet space where your child can retreat when feeling overwhelmed. Use visual schedules or communication tools to help them understand and anticipate transitions, reducing surprises that can trigger stress. Additionally, teaching and practising coping skills, such as deep breathing and mindfulness exercises, can help your child manage their emotions more effectively.

Meltdowns in action

Of course, you won't always be able to prevent a meltdown. Signs of a meltdown in process typically include:

- more intense emotional outbursts, including crying, screaming and yelling
- aggressive behaviour, including hitting, kicking, throwing things and lashing out
- physical distress such as banging their head, stomping feet, clenching fists or jaw and throwing themselves to the ground
- difficulty with communicating, such as an inability to express thoughts and feelings – even becoming non-speaking
- sensory overload, including increased sensory sensitivities to things such as lights and noise
- destructive behaviour such as breaking or throwing things and damaging property.

If your child is experiencing a meltdown, here are some tips for responding effectively:

- Stay calm (this can be *hard*): attempt to remain confident and composed to avoid escalating the situation.
- Provide space: if possible, remove your child from the overstimulating environment and give them space to de-escalate.

- Use reassuring language: speak in a quiet, gentle tone to reassure them you are there to help, and they are safe – it's usually best not to talk *too* much.
- Implement calming strategies: offer sensory tools or other strategies that you know help them, whether it's deep breathing, their weighted blanket or headphones. One family I work with swears by a bottle of lavender oil their child can sniff from – worth a try!
- Be patient: try to avoid rushing the process and allow them enough time to calm down (as difficult as this may be, particularly if you have people spectating).
- Offer distractions: an iPad, fidget toy or discussions about their special interests may help them to regulate.

Having a response plan ready to go can help reduce the length and severity of the meltdown, as well as support your child's post-meltdown recovery in a safe, supportive and compassionate manner. If you find it hard to stay calm when your kid is melting down (which I can very much relate to), you could even write down these steps on a card that you carry around with you.

When responding to meltdowns, it's equally important to know how *not* to respond. As hard as it can be – again, I get it – try to avoid these reactions:

- Panicking: showing fear or frustration will only increase your child's anxiety and escalate the situation (and *nobody* wants that).
- Anger: yelling or raising your voice will only further agitate and exacerbate the situation.
- Threatening punishment or consequences: this is counterproductive and will increase the stress for your child.

- Making critical or patronising comments or attempting to reason with them: during a meltdown, critical or patronising comments can feel invalidating and may increase your child's feelings of shame or frustration, making it harder for them to regain control. Instead of helping, such remarks can lead to more intense emotional reactions or further withdrawal. In the midst of a meltdown, a child's ability to process and respond to criticism is significantly diminished, so it's essential to approach them with empathy and understanding. Providing calm reassurance and focusing on de-escalation helps create a supportive environment where the child can eventually recover and learn more effective coping strategies.
- Using physical restraint: unless they are at risk of harm.
- Making sudden, threatening movements, or getting in their face or personal space: remember they are in *fight*-or-flight mode.
- Ignoring the situation (like we are advised to do with temper tantrums): hoping a meltdown will resolve on its own is likely to lead to further distress.

Avoiding these responses can help to manage the meltdown more effectively and hopefully lead to a better outcome for your child – and yourself. And if your child is melting down in public, remember that we don't care what judgey Cheryl thinks, because her opinion does not matter to you!

One family I recently worked with had a little girl, Alex, who had recently been diagnosed as autistic at the age of seven. Her parents were just learning about the new diagnosis and what this meant for them and for Alex, who had enormous sensory sensitivities and struggled with any changes to her daily routine. The family wanted to be able to go on trips to places like the zoo with Alex and her two siblings. With an upcoming and long-awaited family holiday planned to visit a theme park, they knew the noise, bright lights and large crowds would create an overwhelming environment for her. They sought my help to figure out how to properly support Alex through the experience.

During our sessions, we worked on strategies to identify impending meltdowns and have appropriate supports ready for Alex. As parents to a newly diagnosed child, they hadn't even realised until that point that the years of Alex having what they had called tantrums were actually meltdowns.

As anticipated, on their first day at the theme park, Alex became increasingly agitated. Her parents now knew the signs, as she began covering her ears and squirming, which led to crying and refusing to move. This quickly escalated to Alex throwing herself on the floor where she began to hit and kick. Her parents now recognised these were the signs of a meltdown and knew they had to act quickly to help Alex calm down. As we had discussed, one parent immediately took her to a quieter area of the theme park. On my advice, they had researched this before they went – it's very important to always be prepared – and had discovered a designated quiet room where the lights were dimmed and the noise was minimal.

Once there, they approached Alex calmly, speaking in a soothing voice, acknowledging her feelings and providing comfort. As we had practised, they used phrases like, 'I see this is really overwhelming for you, and we are here to help you.' They then offered Alex a set of noise-cancelling headphones they had prepacked, as well as her travel-sized weighted blanket and favourite soft toy (a mini Beanie Boo). Alex used these and immediately showed signs of relief. They then provided her favourite snacks and a water bottle. After a few minutes in the quiet room, Alex's parent began talking to her gently about moving back out into the theme park, and offering to bring her back to the quiet room for regular breaks to minimise the stress. By identifying an impending meltdown and acting quickly – providing a calm environment and the sensory tools they knew worked for her – Alex's parents were able to help her recover from the meltdown and re-engage with the theme park at her own pace.

This experience helped Alex's parents develop better strategies for managing sensory overload and affirmed that with the right tools (and preparation, practice and *lots* of patience), they would be able to enjoy family trips together. It is not realistic to expect to prevent every meltdown, so the focus is on learning to minimise and manage them.

Shutdowns

A neurosparkly person may also have a more internalised, muted or silent response to extreme overload or stress, known as a shutdown. You know when your computer does that little spinning wheel of death, around and around and around, and you can't make it work, no matter what you do? Yeah, that's a shutdown. Like a meltdown, a shutdown is an involuntary reaction to being overwhelmed, but it is more similar to the body's freeze response than the fight-or-flight response of a meltdown.

A shutdown often involves a child retreating into themself, making it difficult for them to communicate or engage with their surroundings. Think of it as their battery running flat, so there is no more energy to do a single thing. All they can do is rest and recover, which will hopefully start to recharge their battery.

How to distinguish a meltdown from a shutdown, you might ask? Easy. Judgey Cheryl won't notice the shutdown!

Autistic children experience shutdowns when they are so overwhelmed that they withdraw completely, becoming non-responsive, quiet or retreating to a safe space. It is like their brain is hitting the pause button to avoid further sensory input or emotional stress. Shutdowns in ADHD kids might be less common, but can happen when the child feels overwhelmed by too many tasks, emotions or stimuli, leading them to disengage or become unusually quiet and withdrawn.

If people do notice your child having a shutdown, it's important to respond with confidence and clarity. Briefly explain that your child is experiencing a moment of sensory or emotional overload and that they need space to self-regulate. Emphasise that this is a normal response and not a result of misbehaviour. If appropriate, let them know how they can help – such as giving your child space or minimising noise. Providing this context can help others understand the situation better and ensure that your child's needs are respected without additional stress or confusion. So if you have a child who immediately goes quiet upon entering a noisy social situation, and everyone rushes to ask what's wrong – making things worse – it can be helpful to have an answer ready: 'Nikki just takes a few minutes to settle in when she arrives at a party. So she might want to go and cuddle your beautiful dog first, then she will join in when she is ready.'

One of the beautiful girls I work with, Angela, recently celebrated her first birthday at school, having previously been homeschooled. She was so eager to have a cake at school and to let the other kids know it was her birthday, but the noise of 25 loud kids singing 'Happy Birthday' would undoubtedly send her into a shutdown from the sensory overload. I discussed with her mum that she could contact the classroom teacher and explain that Angela would be bringing cupcakes for everyone but did not want a song sung, and that it was to be a very low-key celebration. When it was time for the cakes to come out, the teacher asked all the students to sit quietly and explained that loud noises hurt Angela's ears because they were very sensitive, so the birthday girl's wish was for everyone to sit and eat cupcakes together on the floor with no songs being sung. She got her birthday wish and could not have been happier!

Triggers

Like with a meltdown, it is crucial you learn to recognise the particular signs of a shutdown for your child, which will allow you to provide appropriate support, create a calming environment and offer comfort without further overwhelming the child – or yourself.

Anything that can cause meltdowns can also cause shutdowns, so let's recap:

* sensory overload: intense or overwhelming sensory stimuli such as loud noises, bright lights or strong smells
* emotional overwhelm: high levels of stress, anxiety or emotional distress
* unexpected changes or disruptions to your child's routine or environment

- social overload: overwhelming social interactions or situations with too many people
- physical discomfort: being hungry, tired, thirsty or otherwise uncomfortable
- difficulty communicating: having trouble expressing their needs, leading to frustration.

Shutdowns are still a very common occurrence for Chloé, even at the age of 27. The good thing is, I am now a seasoned professional and can anticipate pretty much any and all scenarios that will lead to a shutdown – and believe me, I am well prepared for every eventuality. For Chloé, some of the most common triggers include:

- any big event, including birthdays and Christmas
- a concert
- speaking at a conference or large event
- wearing an incredibly uncomfortable outfit in an incredibly uncomfortable setting.

Early warning signs

There are a few signs a shutdown might be imminent, and while they are different for everyone, these include:

- Increased withdrawal: your child may become noticeably quiet, retreating from interactions and isolating themselves.
- Avoidant behaviour: they may avoid eye contact, turn away from others or disengage from activities.
- Difficulty communicating: they may struggle to find the words; speak in a flat, monotone or quiet voice; or stop speaking all together.

- Physical signs: they may show signs of physical discomfort, irritability or fidgeting.
- Reduced response to stimuli: they may have a diminished reaction to the environment or even fail to respond to their name, as if they cannot hear you.
- Staring or blank expression: often they will glaze over with a stare or blank expression, which can indicate they are so overwhelmed they are shutting down.

Recognising the early signs of a shutdown can help you prevent the situation from escalating. As with meltdowns, these can include sticking to a predictable routine to provide a sense of security; giving your child sensory breaks in a calm, quiet space; using visual schedules or communication tools to help them understand and anticipate transitions, reducing surprises; and teaching and practising coping skills, like deep breathing and mindfulness exercises, to help your child manage their emotions more effectively.

Shutdowns in full effect

Once a shutdown really gets going, the signs may include:

- reduced communication, including being completely silent or unable to speak
- withdrawing and wanting to hide away and be alone, avoiding eye contact and becoming unresponsive
- difficulty engaging with situations, including having no energy or motivation
- decreased movement, including becoming very still or even frozen and unable to move

- other physical signs, including changes in posture – in particular, curling up, hiding, increasing stimming or covering their face or body
- blank stare, staring into space or having a glazed look.

Some tips for what to do include:

- Provide space: allow your child the time and space to recover without pressure or demands.
- Stay calm: be composed, gentle and reassuring.
- Reduce sensory input: dim lights, lower noise levels and remove any other potential stressors or remove them from the overstimulating environment.
- Offer comfort: empathise, be kind and offer their weighted blanket or favourite snuggle toy, to help them change into sensory-friendly comfortable clothes or PJs, to hop in the bath or shower or to put on their 'safe' TV show or movie (you know, the one they watch on repeat).
- Be patient: your child will need time to process and recover, so do not rush them back to 'normal' activities.

And I also have advice on how *not* to respond to a shut-down, as these actions may prolong or worsen the situation. Please don't:

- push them to just 'snap out of it'
- force interactions or overwhelm your child with questions or probing for details
- ignore their needs or fail to address their comfort
- use harsh or loud language, reprimands, threats, negative comments or ultimatums

- touch them, unless they give you permission to do so
- leave them unless they tell you to go.

Hopefully by following the advice above, you'll be able to support your child and help get their operating systems back up before too long.

COMMUNICATION CARDS

Communication cards are an awesomely simple tool every neurodivergent person needs in their toolbox. They can be especially useful with kids.

These cards contain short phrases, pictures or symbols that can be used to express feelings ('scared', 'overwhelmed'), thoughts ('too many people', 'too much light') or needs ('more space', 'my plushie', 'a hug'). They can be exceptionally helpful for neurodivergent people to use when they are having difficulty speaking, particularly during a meltdown or shutdown. There are lots of free printable cards online, or you can make your own and laminate them, or lots of online stores sell variations of them. The cards can help your child find their voice and independence wherever they are.

Burnout

You may have heard of burnout through your workplace. Sadly, with so much on everyone's plates, it feels like more and more people are burning out these days. Burnout simply describes a state in which a person is no longer able to cope with situations that they previously handled.

Neurodivergent people live in a world that was not made for us. This means we are constantly struggling to meet the neurotypical expectations placed on us, which puts us at a higher risk of burnout. Some research even suggests neurodivergent burnout is a totally distinct condition from the more common type.

Neurosparkly kids are certainly not immune from experiencing burnout. It's useful to know how burnout might look in your child and what steps you can take to support their recovery.

Signs of burnout

Most of the research on neurodivergent burnout comes from autism, but the signs can be similar for kids with ADHD or dyslexia, especially those who attempt to mask their neurodivergent traits to avoid unwanted attention.

Neurodivergent burnout tends to be a longer-term condition, usually happening for at least three months, and can look like:

- Chronic exhaustion: this is not just the regular *big day of school* kind of tired, where they seem refreshed by the next morning. I'm talking *dragging themselves out of bed and having no energy for their special interests* kind of tired.
- Loss of skills: your child might start losing the ability to speak (if they speak to begin with), or start to suffer memory loss or brain fog.
- Changes in sensory sensitivity: this can go either way, with kids becoming either more or less sensitive to sensory inputs (bright lights, loud noises, smells or tastes).

- Emotional dysregulation: they may have more meltdowns and shutdowns, or show increased anxiety.
- More rigid or inflexible thinking: they may become more restricted in the foods they will eat or insist more strongly on following routines.
- Sleep disruptions: your child may sleep much more or much less.

Now, you might be thinking, 'My kid has these symptoms every day!' and, trust me, I hear you. But burnout will usually feel like a whole new level of symptoms, especially when they continue for a longer period.

Recovery from burnout

Once you've realised that your child is in burnout, it's so important that you support them in every way you can to be their authentic neurodivergent selves. This will reduce the load on them trying to meet those unrealistic expectations coming from the outside world and put them on the road to recovery. Some tips include:

- Adjust the schedule: reduce the number of activities and commitments to allow more downtime. Focus on quality over quantity, ensuring your child has ample time for relaxation and self-care.
- Create a calming routine: establish a daily routine that includes predictable periods of rest and low-stimulation activities. This helps your child regain a sense of stability and control.
- Encourage self-care: teach and encourage self-care practices such as deep breathing, mindfulness or engaging

in calming hobbies. These practices can help manage stress and promote relaxation. When Chloé is feeling burned out, I get out her beading kits and mindfulness colouring books, and she enjoys doing some art and craft. For her, it's the ultimate repetitive mindfulness that encourages relaxation.

- Monitor sensory inputs: be mindful of sensory overload. Adjust the environment to minimise overwhelming stimuli and provide sensory breaks or tools that help your child self-regulate.

- Communicate openly: talk to your child about their feelings and experiences. Validate their emotions and work together to identify stressors and develop coping strategies.

- Reintroduce interests gradually: once your child is feeling better, slowly start up their favourite activities again. Ensure these activities are balanced with rest and adapt to their current needs and energy levels.

- Seek professional support: consider consulting with a therapist who specialises in neurodivergent children and can offer tailored strategies and support for managing and recovering from burnout.

- Foster a supportive environment: create a home environment that feels safe and nurturing. Encouragement and understanding from family can significantly impact recovery and wellbeing.

- Encourage sleep: create calming bedtime rituals to encourage more restful sleep. Many parents swear by melatonin for their neurodivergent kids, and it's worth chatting to your doctor or paediatrician about it. There are different types of melatonin, so it may be worth trialling a few to see which one best suits your child.

- Ask for accommodations: perhaps they'll need a reduced workload at school or even a complete break from school for a certain period – take the time to understand your child's needs and be their best advocate.

It can take neurodivergent people more time to recover from burnout (thanks, overstimulated nervous system) so be patient – and make sure you look after yourself, too. Call on your community to allow you to take time out to recharge your own energy supplies. The last thing your child needs is for you to burn out, too.

If the above supports don't seem to be making a difference, or your child is getting worse by the day, don't hesitate to seek professional help (see the resources at the end of the book).

One of the young girls I work with, Lily, who loved school and was bright, creative and intelligent, started showing signs of burnout from her daily school routine. At first, she loved learning new things and interacting with classmates. However, over time, she became overwhelmed by the constant sensory demands of a noisy classroom, the unpredictability of social interactions and the pressure to keep up with assignments. Lily started coming home in tears, exhausted, and her usual enthusiasm for her favourite activities (drawing and reading) waned. She became withdrawn, her anxiety increased, and she frequently complained of headaches and stomach-aches. Despite still saying she loved school, attending five days a week was becoming a real struggle.

Realising that Lily was experiencing burnout, her parents asked for advice on how to deal with it. I worked with the school to encourage the teachers to create a more supportive school environment, arranging for sensory breaks throughout the day and an adjustment to her workload to make it more manageable – including no homework to be sent home. We also negotiated with the school to take Wednesdays off for the foreseeable future, to allow Lily to have a full day's break in the middle of the week. These changes helped Lily begin to recover, showing that understanding her needs and making necessary adjustments were key to supporting her wellbeing and helping her thrive at school. Remember, mental health is more important than *anything*.

Q & A

Q: MY CHILD HAS FREQUENT MELTDOWNS, AND I FEEL SO HELPLESS. I DON'T KNOW WHAT CAUSES THEM AND I DON'T KNOW HOW TO RESPOND. HOW CAN I SUPPORT MY CHILD WITHOUT FURTHER ESCALATING THE SITUATION?

A: Firstly, it's so important to understand meltdowns are not tantrums or misbehaviour; they are intense reactions to feeling overwhelmed. For a neurodivergent child, sensory overload, changes in routine or emotional stress can be much harder to process, leading to a meltdown when they've reached their limit. Some strategies for handling meltdowns include: staying calm and present, reducing sensory overload, avoiding punishment or threats of punishment, helping them co-regulate, preparing for next time and respecting recovery time. Remember, meltdowns are a form of communication from your child, signalling that something is too much for them to handle in that moment. With practice, patience and understanding, you can help them build skills to manage their emotions, while also offering the safety and support that they need.

Q: WHY DOES CHLOÉ GO TO SO MANY CONCERTS WHEN SHE KNOWS THEY WILL LEAD TO A SHUTDOWN?

A: It's quite simple! Because she does not want to miss out on the things she loves – going to see Harry Styles in concert will always outweigh the potential negative consequence of a shutdown afterwards. Understanding that it is imminent and expected allows us to better support Chloé and create an environment that will minimise stressors.

It is crucial for neurodivergent children to engage in activities they love, even if they can sometimes be overwhelming. These passions can offer immense joy and a sense of accomplishment, helping to build confidence and providing a valuable outlet for expression. While it's important to balance these activities with appropriate breaks and supports, allowing your child to pursue their interests enriches their lives and promotes a sense of normalcy. By finding ways to adapt or manage potential stressors, you can help ensure that their experiences remain positive and fulfilling, reinforcing that their passions are worth embracing despite occasional challenges.

To prepare for a likely shutdown, there are a few things we do. If we are away from home, we pack a travel kit of super-comfy clothes, sensory aids and makeup wipes. So many people will see our girl at a concert dressed in her festival outfit, which usually consists of a rainbow of sequins dipped in glitter with brightly coloured eye makeup and knee-high heeled boots. What they won't see is that after the concert, before we are even out of the carpark, these clothes have been pulled off and replaced with an oversized fleecy tracksuit, and the makeup wipes have already removed every ounce of glitter and neon-green eyeshadow. The noise-cancelling headphones are on and the weighted blanket is covering her.

On the way *to* the concert we will have been streaming the current album on repeat and at top volume – singing and dancing to it in the car is an absolute must. On the way *home* from the concert, however, we require silence. And sleep.

When we get home, Chloé goes straight to the bedroom with a cup of tea, favourite snacks and *Bluey* on repeat. Oh and a *do not disturb for at least 48 hours* sign on the bedroom door.

Chapter 4

Family life

Raising your little bear cubs can be difficult and overwhelming at the best of times – managing family dynamics, balancing expectations, ensuring there is time for yourself, your partner (if you have one) and each of your children. It's no wonder we can often feel exhausted. Sometimes as a parent you're like a ringmaster in a circus – while one person is walking a tight-rope, another is standing next to roaring lions, and in among it all there is a funny little clown with oversized shoes, mismatched clothing and hair that hasn't been brushed in days juggling fire, oblivious to what is going on ... while also honking an enormous horn. And you, the ringmaster, are standing in the centre of the big top, just hoping to get through the show in one piece, smiling at the spectators, pretending everything is normal and fine, thinking, *we have to do this same show tomorrow and the day after and then the day after that and oh my gosh I just need a prosecco and a lie down.* One of my favourite sayings is 'not my circus, not my monkeys', which I say to remind people if they are worrying about somebody else's problems that don't involve them. However, today this *is* your circus and they *are* your monkeys. so let's step right up to the greatest show on earth.

Setting your family culture

One thing the ringmaster is responsible for is setting the overall vibe for the daily performance. As parents, we're responsible for setting the vibe, or culture, for our family. We do this with a mix of role-modelling and talking with each other about the expectations we have of our family members. My family now has two neurodivergent parents and (at least!) three neurodivergent kids as well as two neurotypical ones, plus their partners. While this can lead to squabbles as we try to meet everyone's unique needs, our family culture revolves around a few key beliefs – kindness, love, openness and respect – which we apply to every family member. This means leading by example and creating a space where everyone feels heard and valued. It's about embracing differences, showing empathy and being curious about each other's experiences. Openness invites honest conversations, even about difficult topics, while respect ensures each family member's boundaries and needs are honoured. By modelling these values consistently, you cultivate an environment where your child feels safe to be themselves, fostering emotional growth and building lasting healthy relationships both within and beyond the family.

As always, ensure that all you do is neuro-*affirming* not neuro-*damaging* (see the definitions on pages 9–10). Don't say to your kids, 'People don't want to hear about sharks all day, every day. You need to talk about something else.' Instead, you could say, 'Guess what?! I have found someone else who is as interested in sharks as you are – in fact, I think they love them as much as you do!' and present them with books/documentaries/questions about their special interests. Then gather the rest of the family to read, watch or chat with your child about them.

The love language of most neurodivergent kids is sharing their special interest. By valuing their deep interests and giving them opportunities to share them with the rest of your family – and, from there, the world – you will encourage their curiosity and desire to learn. I can also absolutely *guarantee* you will learn some pretty cool stuff in the process. Did you know sharks will go through up to 30,000 teeth in a lifetime? And Liam and Niall from One Direction both had the same middle name – James? And the word velociraptor means 'speedy thief'? Don't say I wasn't listening!

Creating a safe home

Creating a safe home is arguably the most important thing any parent can do for their child. But if you have a neurosparkly child who finds the whole outside world unsafe, overstimulating, scary, unaccepting and just all too much, a calm home – where they have a safe place and unconditional love and acceptance – is an absolute must.

Physically a safe home can include:

* soft and diffused warm lighting (never fluoro or 'noisy' lights – light dimmers are great)
* turning off appliances that tick, rattle or hum
* neutral, soft, pastel colours: nothing too bold or bright or 'noisy' (unless, of course, it's sequins and glitter!)
* no clutter, to minimise sensory overwhelm
* soft rugs or flooring, to tone down floorboards that can echo and magnify noise
* lots of comfort items such as bean bags, big cushions, soft blankets, sensory-friendly furniture

- a dedicated calming space, which may include a tent with fidget toys for self-regulation and favourite soft teddies
- a place to hyperfocus on strong special interests (there is no shame in an entire room in your house being dedicated to your kid's Lego creations or incredible collection of *Titanic* artefacts (or maybe even a Lego creation of the *Titanic*)
- smells that don't overwhelm the senses (try soft diffusers with natural oils)
- routines and charts: a basic morning and evening routine schedule plus a daily reminder of what's on for that day – and what's for dinner – can be so helpful
- sensory-friendly clothing: oversized super-snuggly hoodies or Oodies can work well
- noise-cancelling headphones.

Emotionally a safe home can include:

- Encouraging everyone's passions and strengths by giving them the time to follow them, listening to them and joining in, which shows them they matter. I have learned so many incredible cool facts from the kids I work with. When I was showing one little girl that one of our horses had one blue eye and one brown eye, she looked at me and said, 'Don't you mean he has *heterochromia*?' 'Well, yes, that's *exactly* what I meant!' I replied as I went off to google this word. Did I mention neurosparkly kids are quite simply the smartest and most interesting kids in the world?
- Providing consistency. When your child knows what to expect from you, they are much more likely to feel secure and have the ability to self-regulate with you and see home as their safe place. Prepare everyone for change, using

visuals to highlight changes where possible. Even for me, routine and consistency are so helpful. Every single day I take our dog for the same walk around the block. The kids know, the dog knows and I know . . . rain, hail or shine, we go for a walk. If for some reason I can't, the whole day is thrown into disarray – for me and the dog!

CREATING CONSISTENCY

A few things we did and still do to create consistency include:

- Meals are at 6 pm every night, and everyone sits at the table without devices to chat as a family.
- We have had 'fish and chip' Friday for as long as I can remember. Even the big kids still come home for this one!
- Theme nights, such as Taco Tuesday – the kids find comfort in knowing what these days will bring.

Sibling dynamics

Ah, sibling relationships . . . you can choose your friends but not your family, hey? Most siblings have ups and downs, good days and bad days, times when you would kill them and also times you would kill for them. It is *totally* normal for siblings to fight and have days where they don't get along. But in my experience, many siblings of neurodivergent kids – and, actually, siblings of any kids with additional needs – are among the most kind, caring, compassionate, tolerant, beautiful humans to exist. Of course, it can also be hard for them and natural for them to feel angry, sad, jealous, confused or anxious.

Sibling relationships are often complicated, but they can be even trickier when one (or more) child's needs consistently take precedence. As parents, we have to constantly juggle everyone's needs, which can be difficult when we only have twenty-four hours in a day. We like to think we keep it all even, with no favouritism, but we all know the squeaky wheel gets the oil – and let's be honest, our neurodivergent kids can be pretty squeaky at times.

While we must acknowledge that the squeaky wheel needs oil, we should also keep in mind that the quiet wheels can still seize up or fall off if they are never oiled. So we must make time to meet the needs of all of our little wheels.

Siblings will often be the longest lasting and most important relationships a person can have, so fostering a positive environment and acknowledging that everyone has their own individual needs met is crucial for the sibling relationship to continue developing.

It is important that every day, when you can, you have a one-on-one conversation with each of your children, to check in and see how they are going. This can be just a minute or two while you are in the car on the way home from school, washing the dishes together or saying goodnight. Having set questions for your children creates consistency, and while it may feel structured and formal, it gives them an opportunity to have their voice and feelings heard.

For example, you may ask the same three questions every single evening:

- What made you smile today?
- What made you sad today?
- Is there anything I can do to make tomorrow better for you?

Your children will come to appreciate this short time when they can be heard. Even if you are super busy or away, it only takes a minute or two, and maybe one day you may be lucky enough that your child will ask you these same questions.

Neurodivergent kids sometimes struggle with alexithymia, or difficulty with recognising or describing their feelings. This can make emotions feel overwhelming or confusing, leading to frustration or withdrawal. This does *not* mean they are emotionless – in fact, they're quite the opposite. It just means many of our kids may need extra support to understand what they are feeling.

Parents can help by offering gentle prompts like the questions above; over time this helps to build emotional awareness. Because of this, as your children get older, they will be better able to articulate their true feelings and let you know what is bothering them. It is important to allow them this space to be honest about their feelings, even if those feelings are directed towards their sibling – encouraging them to vent and be open about their frustrations in confidence gives them the opportunity to feel heard.

These check-ins can also be used as teachable moments. For example, when we ask our child, 'What made you sad today?' it may be that their sibling has done something that has upset or angered them. This is an opportunity to work with your child on problem-solving rather than fixing the problem yourself. It may also be a good time to explain some of the needs of their sibling.

If your children share a bedroom, it may help to put rules in place if they have conflicting needs – say, one child is super neat while the other is really messy. Accommodating both needs can be difficult, particularly in shared spaces. I worked with one family who put tape down the middle of the room, and the children were not allowed to set foot or allow a single item to cross that line (or even *breathe* in the general direction of their sibling). Putting up a physical barrier such as shelves or a curtain to divide the room can be helpful, too. Labelling drawers and sections of wardrobes for each child can assist in giving children independence and their own space, and also encourage them to put their things away. This can be helpful in shared bathrooms as well – giving hooks and drawers to each child makes them more aware of their own space and less likely to touch their siblings' things.

When we were foster parents, we had a rule that each child had collections of their 'own' things and their own space, and then there were shared items that were kept in common areas. Teaching kids to understand that each person has their own special items they don't want to share is an important and valuable lesson, particularly important for kids who have extreme attachments to objects.

In our family of five kids, spending one-on-one time with each child can be challenging, so we have always scheduled dates with the kids, where one parent takes one child out. It could be as simple as a play in the park or a cheap McDonald's ice cream, or as fancy as a trip to the theatre or a concert. You can find windows of opportunity every day. It might be keeping one child up after the others have gone to bed to play a board game or watch their favourite show with a bucket of popcorn. Or it could be a sneaky date after you have dropped one child off to piano practice. Intentionally find opportunities to spend one-on-one time with each of your kids, however it works, and make sure they all know you have reserved a spot in your calendar to spend time with them – this helps with sibling rivalry, as they do not need to compete for your attention.

Every week I used to take my eldest son to his hour-long jiujitsu lesson. Being half an hour's drive from home, it was too far to return home during the lesson, so instead I would take my youngest daughter with me and we would find fun things to do in this time. She absolutely loves drawing, so some weeks it was just sitting in the car drawing together, which she loved as much as the times we would go find a great restaurant to have a quick meal. It's the little things!

Saving time for your partner – and yourself

Having two committed parents in a relationship, while not always possible, certainly makes the job easier. If you are in this situation, let me give you my most important tip to sustain this: have a date night at least once a week. If you cannot physically go out without the kids, do something together at home – grab some takeaway with your favourite bottle of wine, watch a movie with some ice cream or play a board game by the open fire. It doesn't need to be expensive or elaborate. It is just a matter of connecting and being able to talk with each other without the constant interruption of your little darlings. The golden rule we always had was no talking about the kids. Find other things to talk about, like, say, each other? You may even remember why you fell in love with them in the first place . . .

Sometimes our kids will try to make us feel guilty for doing something without them. We need to talk to our kids about the importance of parents spending time together alone and explain that this helps keep our family strong. As our big kids have gotten older, they have frequently spoken about how much they love and admire the relationship we have, and how they now strive for it themselves. They also acknowledge how wonderful and important it was (and still is) for us to go out as a couple. In fact, the most common gift our big kids buy us now for birthdays and Christmas are vouchers for beautiful restaurants, which are always so appreciated. It doesn't always have to be dinner, either, often for us it can be as simple as taking the dog for a walk around the block in the evening without anyone following us.

If you are single and raising kids by yourself, alone time is harder to find but even more important. This is where you need to gather a village around you, if you can, and rely on them to mind the kids while you take some breaks. Find a friend you can spend quality time with or schedule alone time for a relaxing child-free bubble bath, massage or whatever you like. Schedule these things in your calendar and prioritise them. Let your kids know this is what you are doing, and why it is so important – don't be ashamed to put your oxygen mask on first.

Encouraging independence

The home environment is the perfect place for neurodivergent kids to practise doing things independently. This requires patience and structure, and involves making routines clear and predictable. Start by breaking down tasks into simple manageable steps, using visual schedules or step-by-step checklists for daily activities to make each task easier to follow. Gradually introduce more responsibility, allowing them to make choices and take ownership of their daily activities, then adjust as needed.

Many parts of self-care can require significant executive functioning skills, which can cause overwhelm for neurodivergent kids. Luckily, there are a growing number of fantastic sensory-friendly items designed to help make self-care easier, and the options are getting better every day. No matter what self-care support you need, there are likely to be things designed to help.

SENSORY-FRIENDLY SELF-CARE

Instead of:	Use:
standard hair brush	tangle-free hair brush
pads or tampons	period underwear
traditional toothbrush	U-shaped sensory toothbrush
mint toothpaste	fruit/bubblegum/flavourless toothpaste
standard dinner plate	divider plate (so the food doesn't touch)

Visual aids are also useful to remind kids of what needs doing. We would often write hygiene schedules on the bathroom mirror with whiteboard markers. Remembering to brush your hair and your teeth is so much easier when the reminder is literally staring you in the face!

Making decisions can be really difficult for our neurodivergent kids, causing elevated levels of stress. One of the biggest battles can be the first decision of the day – what am I going to wear? This can cause total overwhelm and even meltdown or shutdown (see pages 67–81) as kids attempt to make what should be a simple decision. Often, the more options they have, the harder it is to choose. The best way to support our kids is to give them two choices. So, every morning, you could identify two possible outfits suitable for the day's plans, leave them out and let your child choose which one they are wearing that day.

This gives them choice and autonomy but makes it easier for them than picking from their entire wardrobe.

Another brilliant way to encourage independence is involving every child – regardless of their needs or diagnosis – in household chores. This will give them the feeling of being included, valued and essential to the family's functioning. Keep in mind, of course, they are children, so close enough sometimes has to be good enough (I have to remind myself of this constantly!).

The chores can be adjusted to the needs of the child. For example, autistic children with sensory sensitivities may not be able to wash dishes but may be great at sorting the cutlery drawer or matching odd socks (where on earth do they all go, anyway?).

NEURODIVERGENT-FRIENDLY CHORES

When assigning chores to neurodivergent kids, it's essential to consider their strengths, interests, sensory sensitivities and their need for structure. Tasks with clear steps and a predictable routine are likely to work best, such as sorting laundry by colour and family member, feeding the pets or setting the table.

Visual schedules and checklists can help break tasks into manageable parts, making them less overwhelming. For example, instead of simply saying 'go clean your room', and getting frustrated when you find them sitting on the bedroom floor, totally overwhelmed with where to start, I find it best to write down all the steps, like this:

- Put all your dirty clothes in the laundry.
- Put all your clean clothes away (in their labelled drawers/tubs).

- Put all your rubbish in the rubbish bin.
- Bring all your dirty dishes to the sink.
- Put all your toys in the correctly labelled tubs.
- Put all your coloured pencils back in the pencil case.
- Make your bed.
- Put all your shoes in your shoe basket.
- Open your blind and your window for some fresh air.

This is so helpful, even for myself as an adult with ADHD. I also tell my kids to put a line through or tick off each task as they go. It's such a great feeling ticking chores off, and it also helps kids who may find a whole list overwhelming to focus in on one step at a time.

Repetitive chores such as watering plants or vacuuming can be soothing for some kids (as long as they have headphones on while vacuuming), while organising tasks such as putting away toys or arranging books (especially by colour/author/size/genre) can offer a sense of control and accomplishment.

One of my young clients loves nothing more than raking the paddock and picking up horse poo when she comes for equine therapy sessions. Her mum was amazed to see it, and she now earns pocket money keeping their garden clean and tidy, and picking up after their dog. She says it makes her feel calm. Interestingly, in Japan Zen Buddhists rake sand in stone gardens as a meditative act. The simplicity and repetitiveness of this experience can be powerful yet so calming.

Most importantly, celebrate progress no matter how small, and adapt chores to fit each child's unique needs and capabilities.

Food

It is common for neurodivergent people to have unusual eating behaviours, including eating an extremely narrow range of foods. This may be due to sensory issues such as being particularly sensitive to the texture, look, smell, taste and sound of foods. Many autistic people, for example, have very limited diets – it is not unusual for them to survive solely on 'white foods' (chicken nuggets, plain pasta and chips), causing great anxiety in their caregivers. Ritualistic eating behaviours – for example, no foods can touch or be mixed – are also extremely common. The social aspects of eating can be particularly challenging, with sitting at a table with others, using cutlery correctly and waiting for others to finish often inducing additional anxiety.

First up, it can be helpful to rule out medical problems. There is a correlation between gastrointestinal problems and neurodivergence, and many neurodivergent people report being sensitive to gluten and dairy, so your child may be avoiding foods due to gastrointestinal distress. This can be ruled out by a good holistic doctor or naturopath. Seeking out a neuro-affirming dietician who has a good understanding of neurodivergent eating can also be a helpful place to start.

Most neurosparkly children thrive on routine, so embrace regular times for meals. Eating meals as a family at the dining table, where possible, can also be helpful. Often when a child watches others try things, while having choice and control over what they eat, they are more likely to try something new. Having casual conversations and not focusing on food intake can be a helpful and welcome distraction. Involving the kids in preparing the meals and setting the table may also encourage them to try out new foods.

If none of these options are working, however (and we've all been there), feel free to try your child's favourite hobbies as a distraction. You might find that if you pop a plate of food out while they're reading, painting or making Lego, they will mindlessly nibble on it.

Anyone who has ever come to our house for dinner knows there is always an abundance of help-yourself food in the middle of the table – I think feeding people must be one of my love languages. But I also recognise the importance and complication of food, particularly when dealing with eating disorders and neurodivergence and everything in between. Very early on I came to the conclusion that it was easier to have a variety of help-yourself options than rely on a set dish that may not suit everyone. No one wants World War Three at every meal time, and there is nothing worse than spending time (and money) making an incredible meal only to be told 'this is *disgusting*!' (Did I mention honesty is also a very common trait of neurodivergent people?)

New people to our home are always pleasantly surprised and/or shocked at the variety and abundance of food I prepare. They usually think I have made an extra-special effort and over-catered for them as guests, but this is something I have always done. Having a big family with five kids who are always having their friends over, frequent visitors who are often unexpected but always welcome, and years of fostering children as well as one child being vegan, one being vegetarian, one a carnivore and catering for food sensitivities and everything else, it actually makes my life easier. By offering various choices, your child can have autonomy over the food they eat, which can make a big difference in their willingness and enthusiasm to try new things.

I want to make clear that having a 'smorgasboard' of food every night, as I do, does not have to be fancy, elaborate or expensive. Even making a few simple budget-friendly options available, such as a bowl of plain pasta, boiled potatoes, some sliced fruit and chopped salad options, plus a basic meat and protein alternative, increases your chances of everyone finding something they'll eat. Or, if choosing from too many options increases anxiety in your child, you could offer limited choices. You could ask them, 'Would you like chicken or fish for dinner?' (you can pretend you're at a wedding or on an aeroplane!).

Be patient, creative and don't let mealtimes become battle-grounds. When Chloé was about five, she went through a period where she did not want to eat fruit. Bananas, in particular, were a sudden no-go. At the same time, she was obsessed with watching a young Bindi Irwin on a wildlife documentary TV series called *Bindi the Jungle Girl*. I remember seeing Bindi eating bananas and talking about how she only eats bananas for breakfast. So we renamed bananas 'Bindi bananas' and talked about how bananas gave Bindi the superpowers to be a wildlife warrior. I am not even kidding when I say from that moment on, every time we went to the supermarket Chloé would *beg* for 'Bindi bananas' and could not get enough of them. When cyclones caused banana prices to skyrocket, I may have momentarily regretted naming them Bindi bananas . . . but I still bought them for her. I still laugh when I hear my now 27-year-old Chloé call them this. Of course, she's back to not liking them again, and she no longer falls for the Bindi banana hype – these days I might have more luck if I rename them Brachiosaurus bananas!

Some other creative ways to make food more exciting for kids include:

- making fun food pictures on plates with the kids (the Japanese do this so well)
- grating veggies to hide them in things such as pasta sauces
- putting extra sustenance – yoghurt, frozen fruit or protein powder – in smoothies
- chopping up lots of foods – fruit, vegetables, rice crackers, cheese, dips – and calling it a 'party plate' (this works for most children, not just the neurodivergent ones)
- 'dinner winner' plates, where you can make eating into a fun game and separate the food so that a special covered treat awaits them when they finish
- making little menus, like they do in hospitals, where kids can tick the foods they want to eat that night – again giving them some autonomy but also making meals fun.

It's important to keep offering a range of foods. Children may have to try a food dozens of times before they decide they like it. And as hard as it is, try not to make a big deal about whether or not your child tries specific foods. Ultimately, as long as they are eating something – even if it's nothing but chicken nuggets and chips – then it is better than nothing. Especially once you have battled an eating disorder.

Make sure you reach out for help immediately if do you suspect your child has an eating disorder (more on this in chapter 6). It is a very serious disease needing immediate support and help. As someone who struggled with eating disorders for years with Chloé, I know how difficult and important this is.

Sleep

I work with so many families who find sleep one of the most difficult issues, as it can be so disruptive for the whole family. Finding what works for your child is the key. Encouraging sleep in neurodivergent kids often requires a structured, calming routine that takes their sensory needs into account. You could try:

- creating a predictable bedtime routine with visual schedules to guide them through all of the steps, such as brushing their teeth, putting on their pyjamas and reading a book
- minimising sensory distractions by adjusting lighting, sound or bedding to match their comfort levels and preferences, using weighted blankets, bed tents or white noise machines if your child finds them soothing
- being consistent, trying to maintain similar bedtimes and wake-up times, even on weekends, if possible.

Giving your child gentle, reassuring support through this routine can help reduce anxiety around sleep and create a sense of safety and relaxation for a better night's rest . . . for everyone.

Sometimes you may need to give yourself permission to try doing things a bit differently. So many autistic children can fall asleep quicker and easier while watching their favourite familiar show – something that parenting 'experts' often advise against can be the very thing that gets your child, and you, a good night's sleep. For us, this was an absolute life-saver. Literally the *only* way we could get Chloé to sleep was when she was watching her favourite movie or show at the time. It became a choice between attempting to get her to sleep for several hours without the TV and having her asleep within minutes of watching her safe show. In this case, the screen time won – sometimes you just have to pick your battles.

One of the girls I work with, Sam, struggled with racing thoughts and sensory overload at bedtime. Her little ADHD brain would come alive at night, making it so hard for her to wind down and get ready for sleep. I worked with her parents on introducing a calming, repetitive bedtime routine, using strategies such as deep breathing exercises and meditation (there are so many simple kids meditations for free on YouTube), and incorporating a sensory-friendly environment that included blackout curtains, a bed tent to make her feel safe and enclosed (these are so much fun and can be found cheaply online), and a soft, textured blanket. We found a 'sleep spray' (a bottle of water with some lavender oil in it), which her parents sprayed in her room and bed to help her associate the smell with it being time for sleep. They incorporated a visual timer to signal the countdown for when it was time to start the transition to bed. After a few weeks of consistency, Sam started to fall asleep faster, even staying asleep and in her bed, which she now loved. The structured routine and few additional changes helped Sam associate bedtime with relaxation, greatly improving her sleep quality – and, in turn, that of her parents.

Pets

Pets provide companionship, loyalty and friendship, and can be a wonderful addition to the family, particularly for neurodivergent kids who may struggle with human friendships. Animal companions can help kids develop social, sensory and communication skills and have been shown to be effective in reducing stress and anxiety. A child can learn responsibility by feeding and watering and cleaning up after a pet. (On the practical side, visual schedules, reminders and automatic feeders can be invaluable tools to support the care of an animal and ensure they are not forgotten about.)

Being responsible for the care and happiness of an animal can encourage a young person to look after themselves better, too. One of the young men I work with, Tom, was depressed and housebound and found it hard to even get off the couch. When he got a dog who needed to be walked every day, it made him get up and outside whether he felt like it or not, because he was focused on the needs of his dog. The more he got out and into the fresh air, the more he realised he enjoyed it. This led to him joining a dog socialisation class on the weekends, where he learned about dog obedience, and at the same time began interacting with humans, too. It can be so much easier to engage in conversation with someone when an animal is involved.

We have always had pets, and they are an important part of our family. Where possible, we have tried to allow each of our kids to have the individual pets they wanted to have, and we have found the benefits far outweigh the negatives. The only time I would draw the line is if my kids asked for a pet snake, as I am *terrified* of them – thankfully none of them ever have!

Probably my favourite story of pet ownership is about our son who as a preschooler announced he wanted a 'little pig'. He didn't have an animal of his own at the time, so we thought this was gorgeous and agreed. Having recently purchased land, we decided it would be fun to own a pig. We immediately found someone selling a miniature pig and brought it home for him. In hindsight, I realise he did look a little perplexed when this 'little pig' arrived home in a trailer. As the pig continued to grow and grow and grow, eventually getting to 200 kilos plus, and eating anything and everything in sight (including trying to nibble on its owner's little legs every time he reluctantly entered its pen to feed it), we decided maybe having a (now gigantic) pig was not such a great idea after all, especially as we couldn't keep up with the amount of food it needed.

We reluctantly told our little boy we were going to find a new home for the pig, which he (surprisingly) very happily agreed with. The day the pig went off to his new home, we were expecting tears, but our little boy quietly turned to us and said, 'Mummy, when I said I wanted a little pig, I meant a guinea pig not an *actual* pig.' We laugh about this to this very day. Needless to say, we went straight to the pet shop that afternoon and bought our very happy boy a long-haired *guinea pig*, whom he named Spider-Man (of course!). Spider-Man lived for many, many years, fathering many babies, and was a much better investment than the accidental not-so-miniature pig.

Other (human) relationships

Your immediate family will, of course, not be the only people in your neurodivergent child's life. Grandparents, aunts and uncles and other relatives, family friends and neighbours will all be popping in and out, and some advance preparation can go a long way towards keeping these relationships running smoothly.

Fostering relationships between neurosparkly kids and close relatives can be deeply enriching for both the child and the family. Encourage regular low-pressure interactions that respect your child's sensory needs, communication styles and interests. It might be baking together, playing a favourite game, or watching a movie together – anything that can create positive bonding experiences.

It is so helpful to educate family about your child's unique needs and preferences, allowing them to adjust their interactions accordingly. Use open communication and gradual, supportive introductions that help build trust and affection, strengthen family ties and create a supportive, inclusive environment for the child. You might also find this is a time when you will need to educate people and advocate for your child, especially with some of the older generations, who may have preconceived ideas about neurodiversity or raising children.

One of the families I work with found that their daughter Ava's grandfather didn't understand or support her autism diagnosis, and he was causing a lot of harm when Ava spent time alone with him. Some examples they fed back to me were that he would say things to her like, 'Everyone is being diagnosed autistic these days. You don't seem autistic,' and this was causing a lot of distress. We discussed the importance of putting

Ava's needs and safety above everything, but if they were wanting to foster a positive relationship, they would need to talk to him about it, which they did. They also chose not to leave Ava alone with him, so that he would not get the opportunity to make hurtful or ignorant comments. Sometimes, sadly, you may have to make the choice not to engage with family members who are not safe for your kid – remember their mental health, and yours, comes above everything.

Another of my clients, seven-year-old Henry, who is autistic, was really struggling to connect with his grandparents, who were so eager to have a positive relationship with him like they did with their other grandchildren. Henry's parents were desperate for him to be comfortable with his grandparents, as they were the only people they felt were safe enough to babysit. They were also finding it hard to see that the grandparents were struggling to engage with Henry when a relationship with the other grandkids came so easily.

Together, we worked on some simple strategies Henry's parents could suggest to the grandparents, including having them create a welcoming environment that incorporated his interests (such as building model cars) into their visits. They also provided the grandparents with some simple information and strategies on Henry's sensory preferences and communication style, helping them adapt their approach to him. Gradually, the grandparents began engaging Henry in these activities, which led to meaningful interactions and improved bonding (and Grandpa even found a special new interest, too). Over time, Henry grew more comfortable (and even excited) about spending time with his grandparents, and his parents got to go out knowing their boy was not only safe but happy.

Special events

Life is full of big celebrations. While many people love these special events and look forward to them all year, for neurodivergent people events such as Christmas can be a social and sensory nightmare. There are so many expectations that come with the festivities: that you'll attend large family gatherings; eat and enjoy lots of specific traditional foods; be thrilled with the flashing lights, Christmas decorations and Christmas carols; gratefully and graciously receive gifts from relatives who don't know your special interests; and reciprocate affection – even to stinky-breathed Uncle Joe or judgey Aunty Beryl you see once a year. Ugh!

There are so many things you can do as a parent to support your kids – and yourself – to survive Christmas and other big, exciting life events:

- Know your limits. You simply may not be able to attend each and every event you and your family are invited to. Prioritise those that are most important to you and attend those. You may decide to attend events and leave much earlier than everyone else, or you may choose to catch up with other people at a later date. Or maybe never.

- Communicate your needs to those who may be impacted. For example, you may decide to send an email, text or letter to your parents ahead of time if you know they will struggle with the accommodations your kids need. Outline how much you love the celebration and understand the importance of it to them, but that it is too overwhelming for your child. You can say you either won't be coming at all, and would rather catch up just with them at a later date, or that you will be making some adjustments.

SENSORY KITS

Having a range of items on hand to manage your child's sensory sensitivities when you're out and about can be a real lifesaver. These do not need to be expensive and can often be purchased at discount stores. The following list is a great start, though you'll be able to develop your own as you get to know your child's specific needs better:

- fidget toys: putty, slime, stress balls, pop its, fidget spinners and cubes
- tiny soft toys, like mini Beanie Boos on keychains, can be great to hide inside your pockets or clothing to stroke and fidget with; no one but your child will even know it's there
- noise-cancelling headphones: some kids prefer the over-ear ones, others prefer in-ear
- weighted/sequin/plush blankets: different fabrics appeal to different people, so try a few
- sunglasses and hoodies to minimise exposure to bright light
- loose, soft, comfortable clothing (we love our Kmart tracksuits).

- If your kids *despise* the traditional foods of that celebration (roast turkey, anyone?), do not be afraid to take your own safe foods with you. No one should be forced to eat food they don't like just because it's 'tradition'. Pack a lunchbox with your kids' favourite foods that you can quietly pull out when the big meal is served. If Aunty Beryl starts questioning why your kids aren't eating her famous trifle, simply reply firmly and nicely that your child follows a very specific diet. Aunty Beryl doesn't need to know that the very specific diet is actually chicken nuggets and chips.

- Accommodate sensory sensitivities, especially since these can increase during stressful and anxious times. Experimenting or working with an occupational therapist (OT) can help you identify what may work best for your child. Pack a sensory kit with everything in it that may be helpful. If your child needs to sit in a quiet corner with an iPad, a weighted blanket and earphones, who is it going to hurt?

Travel

Travelling can be a wonderful experience for families. But it can also be an absolute nightmare, especially for those who don't like change. A number of things can make travel easier for us and our kids, including good preparation, keeping to routines and taking familiar things with you.

Role-playing is a another great idea to get your child used to what to expect. My ten-year-old client Abbey was recently going to Europe for the first time, so we role-played how the security people would ask her to stop, put her arms up and get scanned like an x-ray. We spoke about how this wouldn't hurt, and they may even ask Abbey to take her shoes off or scan her body with a wand and her hands up in the air, but her mum or dad would be close by if this happened. We talked about sniffer dogs at the airport, customs people opening Abbey's bags, and having to get her photo taken for passport control. Covering as many scenarios as possible means travel will be more predictable. And we know predictable is usually good.

Making a 'social story' to prepare and explain to your child what to expect in particular social situations is also very helpful. With Abbey, we created a social story that covered absolutely everything: counting down the time until she left, packing her bag for the plane, leaving her home and pets, getting through airport security, what to expect on the plane – down to the fine details of 'ear popping', what take-off and landing feel like, the sound of the engines, possible turbulence, the lights going on and off at different times, going to the toilet and eating meals – plus what differences to expect in the countries she was visiting. Review this story as often as you can building up to the flight so they are as familiar as possible with what to expect. There are so many things we take for granted that need to be explained, and a social story is a great way to do this to settle everyone's nerves. A good OT, if you have one, can help with this. Otherwise, the internet is full of wonderful ideas to create a social story for just about any scenario you need.

SOCIAL STORIES

Not sure where to start with making a social story? Here are some practical tips.

- Select the best format for your child. This might mean a hard copy, using materials such as poster paper, index cards or a small notebook; or going digital, using a template on a computer or tablet.
- Pick a social situation that your child finds challenging, such as going to a birthday party or asking a question in class.
- Write out the story in small, manageable steps, using simple sentences and first-person language to help your

>>>

child connect with the ideas. For example, 'I will walk into the birthday party. It might be very noisy with lots of people.'

- Add pictures to illustrate each step. You can use actual photos of your child or the setting, as well as clip art or drawings. There are apps available to help with creating digital versions.
- Use positive and reassuring language. Highlight what the child may see, hear and experience, with a focus on how they might navigate the situation in a neuro-affirming way. For example, 'If I feel overwhelmed, I can tell an adult. It is okay to take a break.'
- Include your child's name or favourite things in the story to make it more engaging. For example, if they love horses, add them to the visuals or talk about them finding a 'quiet horse corner' to rest.
- Read the story together multiple times before the situation arises. Make it part of your routine so your child knows what to expect and feels prepared.

Create a calendar where they can cross off the days until you go. A physical calendar they can mark off with a pen gives them a concrete and visual way to both prepare for the trip and understand the concept of time. This can also be helpful while you are away to reassure them that they will be returning to their home.

On the plane, take all their favourite snacks as it is likely they will not like or eat the plane food (who does, really?). Taking chewy lollies and gum – even if they are not normally allowed these things – is a good idea to help with settling eardrums and also provide sensory stimulation. Carrying a good range of familiar foods for your child means they won't go hungry. (My husband and second-eldest daughter are the *only* two people in the world I have ever heard of who *love* plane food. Every time one of them travels, they send the other all the photos of their food and rate it . . . weird!)

Packing your child's favourite snuggle toy, blanket and sensory items can be helpful to soothe them and remind them of home. Every time I travelled with my kids when they were young, I would take a bag full of new items I would bring out to surprise them at scattered times throughout the flight, particularly if they were getting bored or anxious. I would stock up on new colouring books, stickers, putty, mini games or toys . . . anything to keep them entertained and distracted. One of the best things I found was those little dinosaur eggs you scrape to find the dinosaur inside. This takes a lot of time and patience, so it's perfect for long flights. Just don't give them everything at once. Having a screen right in front of them with games and entertainment is a great distraction, and something most kids love – especially as we don't give them time limits while travelling.

The Hidden Disabilities Sunflower lanyard program is a great initiative. People with a hidden disability can choose to wear the sunflower lanyard, which discreetly indicates to staff and others that they may need more time, support or understanding. It is an international approach that most airports and airlines are familiar with. It can mean not having to line up in the normal queues and getting first access on and off the plane. Check out the Hidden Disabilities Sunflower website for a list of airlines and airports that support this important program (https://hdsunflower.com/us/insights/post/airports-around-the-world).

Q: HOW DO I MANAGE THE STRESS OF CARING FOR MULTIPLE CHILDREN WITH MULTIPLE NEEDS IN ONE HOUSEHOLD?

A: I have a few tips I give the parents I work with to practise, and these include:

- Relaxation and breathing strategies: set some time aside each day for mindfulness and meditation and learning how to breathe properly. There are so many great apps and websites and information online, and this is something you can do anywhere at any time – even when the three kids are in the back of the car killing each other.

- Gratitude: practising this every day has been proven to improve your wellbeing and mental state. It helps to write down what you are grateful for at the end of the day, and it's a fantastic ritual to practise with the kids. It can be as simple as, 'I am grateful for the rainbow I saw today.'

- Organisation: this can be a hard one, especially if you are neurodivergent yourself, but I promise you it's a huge one for helping you feel like you have things under control. Simple things such as doing your food shopping online weekly instead of running to the shops daily with a tribe of kids, spending a couple of hours on a Sunday meal-prepping for the week, and getting everyone in the household to chip in and help with small daily tasks can ensure you feel more on top of things.

- Scheduling: have a huge family calendar that includes everyone's appointments for the month. I take a bit of time at the start of each month to make sure the calendar is up to date, and as I say to my kids, if it's not on the calendar, it's not happening!

- Routine: predictability is so helpful when you have multiple children with multiple needs, and it can make life so much easier and less stressful for everyone.

Q: MY NEURODIVERGENT CHILD OFTEN FEELS OVERWHELMED AT FAMILY GATHERINGS, AND WE HAVE A LOT OF THEM! HOW CAN I HELP MY CHILD FEEL MORE COMFORTABLE AND INCLUDED AT THESE EVENTS, SO WE DON'T HAVE TO MISS OUT ON THEM?

A: Helping your neurodivergent child feel comfortable at family gatherings involves preparing them – and your family – in advance, and creating a supportive environment at the event itself.

Start by discussing the upcoming event with your child. It may even be helpful to put it on a calendar, so they know it's coming up. Outline what to expect and address any obvious concerns they may have. Use visual schedules or social stories to help them understand the sequence of activities. Communicate openly with family members about your child's needs ahead of time, to ensure your child feels supported and included, whatever this looks like for them.

At the event, offer a quiet space where your child can take breaks, if needed, and provide sensory tools or comfort items they can use. You might also plan for shorter, more manageable visits and include activities that align with their interests to make the experience more enjoyable. Consider getting there before the event starts so they can familiarise themselves with their surroundings and find a safe space for them to set up their own area – a small study or someone's bedroom is an ideal place for this. If the event will be particularly noisy or overwhelming, a small pop-up tent, an iPad and some headphones are great to take with you – plus all their favourite snacks and sensory toys.

Some family members may feel your child needs to be part of all the formalities, but if your child will be happier and safer tucked out of the way, then explain this and leave them to it. That way both you and your child can continue to enjoy family events without the pressure.

Chapter 5

School

School can be a challenging place for neurodivergent kids for so many reasons. Many things at school can cause enormous sensory challenges – from fluorescent lights to echoing gyms, piercing bells, smelly toilets and loud, yelling children. This means your child may end up in sensory overload all day long. Managing homework, school projects and deadlines and preparing for exams can all be difficult for people who struggle with the executive functioning skills of planning and carrying out tasks. Navigating social interactions all day every day, plus rules and expectations that change between classes and teachers, can all be very overwhelming. Some neurodivergent children, particularly autistic ones, struggle with fine and gross motor skills, which are used in school for everything from writing to cutting, painting, jumping, catching and skipping.

Given how much time our kids spend at school, it's critical that their learning environment is helping them thrive, not merely survive. And this is absolutely possible! But first let's take a look at the environment that Chloé barely survived.

Chloé's schooling

Despite being academically ready for Prep – as in, knowing her ABCs and her 123s ('and did you know that a snail can sleep for three years at a time?') – our girl was not *really* ready to start school. Not at five, and not even at fifteen.

Like many young children when they first start school, she was very clingy and teary. She was never excited to go, so every morning there would be tears and tantrums, stomach-aches and headaches, and pleading not to go. She just wanted to stay home with me.

Every day when I walked her to the classroom, the Prep teacher would assure me Chloé would likely stop crying five minutes after I had gone, but every day when I collected her, some 6.5 hours later, she would still be crying hysterically. Needless to say, my heart broke daily. I would walk out of the gate in tears, too, with many a well-meaning fellow parent trying to console me by saying Chloé would stop five minutes after I left, or that she would 'grow out of it'. It got to the stage where teachers would be waiting for my car in the morning to help drag her out and peel her off me, and most mornings both of us would be in tears.

The teachers soon admitted that, unlike other children, Chloé did *not*, in fact, stop crying after I had left. They were unsure what to do with her. I was surprised. As she was a bright girl who loved learning, I had assumed she would love school. But it was clear she hated it.

We tried several different primary schools in the hope we would find one that she liked, but each time it just got worse. She was unable to make friends. She was never invited to a single birthday party, and no one would attend hers. She started to make herself physically sick to avoid school. She could vomit on command and get herself so worked up that she would faint. Many trips to doctors and hospitals, and even a couple of ambulance rides, eventually showed these physical symptoms were a result of anxiety.

As parents, it broke our hearts to see Chloé never invited to a single birthday party and no one ever turning up to hers. So we decided to throw a party that was so wonderful that everyone would want to attend. Yes, we would *bribe* the kids at school to come. Surely that would work! Parenting 101 right there . . . or maybe not.

So for Chloé's tenth birthday, we went all out and hired a stretch limousine to actually pick up all her guests from their houses, so they would *have* to come. Then we took the girls out for shopping and lunch, literally buying their friendship and spoiling them rotten. We spent far more money than we could afford, but if it got her some friends then it would be worth it. They all had an absolute ball, and we thought they were a lovely bunch of girls – our plan had appeared to work. But the very next day at school, not one of them spoke to our child. In fact, they ripped off the 'best friends' matching necklaces we had bought them all and threw them in the face of our broken-hearted girl.

If primary school was bad, secondary was horrendous. Suddenly the gap between Chloé and others of her age seemed to be huge. While the other girls were suddenly into bands and boys, fashion, makeup and hair, ours was oblivious to current trends. She would still rather be reading encyclopedias and learning facts in her own little world. She chose clothes for their comfort – and lack of scratchy tags – over fashion. She would go to school with little pieces of hay stuck in her hair, because she'd forgotten to brush it after feeding her ponies.

It had been kind of okay to be a little different at primary school, but at high school she became the main target of the mean girls. They mocked her for everything from the shape of her eyes to the colour of her hair, and even the size of her feet. They were relentless in their bullying. It wasn't until she was older that we learned the full extent of it. Girls writing threatening notes and leaving them in her locker, daring her to take her own life, calling her the most revolting names and spreading scandalous lies and rumours about her. These girls made life hell for our daughter, despite our daily pleas to the school to make it stop.

In my experience, while many schools state they have an anti-bullying policy and that they strictly monitor it, when it comes to holding the bullies accountable, they tend to look the other way and deny any bullying exists. Girls, in particular, seem to be very clever at not being caught, making life even harder for the child being bullied to prove it is actually happening. The funny thing is so many of these bullies now comment on Chloé's socials, claiming to have been friends with her at school – so I guess Chloé gets the last laugh. It's probably not good as a social worker to say success is the best revenge, but sometimes we are allowed a bit of pettiness when we've seen our kids treated horribly.

If your neurodivergent kiddo is having a similarly rough time of it in a mainstream school, let's walk through the other options, step by step, so you can calmly and confidently approach decisions about school.

Option 1: A neurodivergent-friendly school

I know many neurodivergent kids who absolutely thrive in school, but finding an appropriate school is crucial. Some schools do a much better job than others of catering to neuro-diversity, but in my opinion, even more schools simply pay lip service to doing so. Choose your school carefully and don't be afraid to try something different if it's not working for your child.

Every single day, parents ask my opinion on *this* school or *that* school. My answer is almost always the same: for every person who loves a school, there is another who hates it. Very rarely have I heard of a school that's perfect for everyone. Occasionally I hear of a school that is awful for everyone, and that's the only time I will say 'don't go there'.

Before deciding on which school to send your child to, ask around the local neurodivergent community for recommenda-tions, making a list of which schools are good according to multiple sources and which to avoid. Then go and check them out yourself, and ask all the questions so you can make an informed decision: how they work with neurodivergent kids and others with additional needs, and what supports they offer. Just as the school must make accommodations, and show acceptance and awareness of a child using a wheelchair or a deaf child, so they must with a neurodivergent child.

Many neurodivergent kids thrive in alternative settings such as Steiner, Montessori or Waldorf schools, where there is often an emphasis on outdoor time, loving and respecting nature, using music and story to deliver lessons, and a focus on move-ment and play. These schools seek to nurture the 'whole child' rather than simply focusing on the academic side of things.

Unfortunately they also come with fees so may be out of reach for many families.

Think about the type of school that may best fit your neuro-sparkly child. If you have a girl who mostly plays sport with the boys, an all-girls school is likely to be unsuitable. If you have a child who hates sport, a sport-focused school is not the right one. What is a great school for one won't necessarily be a great school for the next.

Trust your gut when walking around a school. Take your child and trust their gut, too. Talk to teachers, talk to parents, talk to students.

RED FLAGS AND GREEN FLAGS FOR SCHOOLS

Red flags:

- focusing only on academics
- high staff turnover
- school grounds covered in litter or graffiti
- a concrete jungle with no trees or gardens
- library closed at lunchtime
- filthy, stinky toilets
- kids walking around alone, looking miserable.

Green flags:

- kids look happy
- bullying policy happily shared
- willing to accommodate sensory needs and make reasonable adjustments (including to uniform policy)
- kids walking around wearing headphones
- has programs for students above or below expected level
- wellbeing included in the curriculum
- offers subjects your child will want to do (particularly important in high school)

>>>

- shares your religious/philosophical/moral values
- has open communication between the school and the parent
- is an easy and safe commute for your child, knowing they will do this for many years.

Option 2: Schooling from home

Regardless of how much training the teachers have had or how many books they have read about neurodivergent kids, when it comes to really dealing with them, in my experience not a lot of teachers, or schools, truly get it. (Though, like all people, teachers have very different levels of understanding, empathy and tolerance, and a fantastic teacher can make all the difference to your child's experience at school.)

Your child's teachers may report that they are quiet and well-behaved in class, which might be very different from what you see at home. Their behaviour can be misinterpreted as shyness or compliance, but it's often actually a sign that they are expending a tremendous amount of energy to mask their symptoms and fit in at school. By the time they get home, they may be emotionally exhausted from the effort of holding it together all day, which can result in them releasing pent-up stress in the forms of meltdowns or explosive outbursts.

This pattern reflects the immense effort these children put into navigating a neurotypical world. For a child to have to camouflage their true self to fit in with their peers is not only exhausting but also devastating, as they are hiding their authentic self, which can ultimately lead to psychological issues, depression and anxiety (more on this in chapter 6).

Understanding this pattern can help parents and teachers provide the support needed to create safe, calming spaces where children can decompress and express themselves without judgement or added pressure.

Some neurodivergent children may appear disruptive in class, at times, but this behaviour often stems from their unique neurological processing rather than intentional defiance or misbehaviour. Sadly, many teachers fail to see the difference, which can result in detentions, suspensions and even expulsions. For instance, a child with ADHD might call out answers or struggle to sit still, due to impulsivity and a need for movement. An autistic child might make repetitive noises or leave their seat to cope with sensory overload or anxiety. These behaviours are not necessarily due to a lack of interest (although our neurodivergent kids *often* do better learning about topics they love) or respect but may be coping mechanisms or responses to overwhelming stimuli. It is crucial to understand that such disruptions are simply a part of how neurodivergent children experience and interact with the world. With the right support and accommodations – such as sensory breaks, flexible seating and clear and consistent instructions – teachers can help these students manage their needs more effectively, fostering an inclusive and supportive classroom environment for everyone, not just neurodivergent kids.

In our experience, sadly, school was far more damaging than beneficial. After trialling several different schools – public, private, Catholic and everything in between – we came to the realisation that no school was likely going to be the right fit for Chloé.

As Chloé's anxiety and behaviour at school continued to worsen, we began to consider the option of homeschooling – something I had never imagined I would do. To me, homeschoolers were extremists and birdwatchers, who lived in kombi vans and wore weird clothes. One evening after a particularly bad day, our diagnosing psychologist said to me bluntly, 'You either homeschool her or you risk losing your daughter forever. The choice is yours.' That shocked me to the core and was the wake-up call we needed. We made the decision then and there to school Chloé from home, as I just couldn't force her through another day of hell.

She never went back – not even to empty her locker or say goodbye to her classmates (after all, she didn't have a single friend). Her dad went to the school, collected all of her stuff, emptying her locker (and the entire lost property room), and the very next day our schooling-from-home journey began. We applied to Distance Education Victoria, now known as Virtual School Victoria, or VSV, and very quickly we were approved and started.

For us, choosing distance education for Chloé was the best thing we ever did. It meant she was not only safely at home and away from bullies, she was also supported one-on-one with work and had plenty of time to follow her passions, which fuelled her and made her happy.

Distance education vs homeschooling

Whenever I mention the idea of schooling from home to families whose kids are hating school, the first thing they say is, 'I could *never* do it.' And that was my first reaction, too. Parents think it is hard, but I can assure you, if you've been through the horrors of school refusal you will find this a much easier alternative – for both you *and* your child. There are two options available for schooling from home: distance education and homeschooling.

Distance education is where the kids still have teachers who assign and mark their work. In Australia, distance education is available to children who live too remotely to attend a local school face to face, or who fall under a particular enrolment category, such as medical (which can be physical or social and emotional) or working as an athlete or performer, any of which can limit their ability to physically attend a face-to-face school.

Distance education can offer significant benefits for neurodivergent children (besides the obvious one of not making them attend a physical school). Usually it offers a wider range of subject options than a standard school, which can be great for catering to specific interests. It also provides a more flexible and accommodating learning environment than traditional schooling. At home, children can customise their surroundings to minimise sensory overload – reducing the impact of bright lights, loud noises and other distractions that make a school learning environment challenging. Distance education also allows for a more personalised pace, giving students the opportunity to take breaks when needed, revisit challenging material or move quickly through content they find easier (or boring). The flexibility can reduce anxiety and fatigue associated with rigid school schedules, and help children better manage their energy and focus. Learning can be tailored to individual styles, making lessons more engaging and accessible. The adaptability creates a more supportive, less stressful educational experience, enabling them to thrive academically and – more importantly – emotionally, and all while in their PJs and ugg boots, if they wish!

It does mean one person needs to be home with the child, but this responsibility may be shared among parents, friends, grandparents, older siblings, aunts or uncles. Depending on the flexibility of your work, your child may be able to do their schooling alongside your work, or you may be able to work from home. I chose to use the time to do further study alongside Chloé, first doing a double degree in nursing and midwifery then a degree in social work, all while helping Chloé complete distance education – come to think of it, I probably should have got a certificate for that, too!

Obviously there are other things to consider, too, such as having access to reliable internet and a dedicated computer, and your child must be comfortable on and in front of the computer.

Distance education can be an excellent way to prepare students for the self-directed learning style of university. By fostering independence, time management and self-advocacy skills, distance learning encourages students to take greater responsibility for their own education, which is crucial for success in higher education. Distance education allows students to navigate online learning platforms, communicate with teachers virtually and manage their study schedules, all of which are common in current university settings. Additionally distance education emphasises project-based learning and critical thinking, helping students develop the ability to research, plan and execute assignments independently. This flexibility and autonomy can build confidence and adaptability, equipping students with the tools needed to handle the less structured environment of university life. I have spoken to a number of university lecturers who have said they can identify the students in their class who have been distance education students.

Depending on where you live and the availability of distance education, there are different requirements for acceptance. Check out the resources on pages 289–90 for more information.

Homeschooling, on the other hand, typically involves developing and following your own curriculum. Homeschooling can be a beneficial option for neurodivergent children because it offers a flexible and tailored learning environment that meets their unique needs. For many families, it provides the opportunity to create a pace and structure that aligns with their child's interests, strengths and sensory needs, free from the pressure of traditional school systems. This can be especially helpful for children who struggle with overstimulation, social challenges or rigid routines in conventional school settings. Parents can integrate therapeutic supports such as sensory breaks or movement-based learning into their daily schedule, fostering a more neuro-affirming approach to education. While homeschooling requires careful planning and commitment, the ability to adapt lessons to a child's learning style often leads to more meaningful engagement and less burnout, both for the child and the family.

One of my clients, Ethan, an eight-year-old autistic boy, had struggled for three years in mainstream school. The constant noise, bright lights and unpredictable social interactions left him overwhelmed and anxious. His meltdowns became more frequent, he was always in trouble at school, and his parents noticed he was losing interest in learning altogether. Even with multiple accommodations in place, the school environment was simply not working for him.

Ethan's parents decided to try homeschooling. They set up a calm, predictable environment that reduced his sensory overload, and his lessons were adapted to his interest in Lego. His mum was able to incorporate regular sensory breaks and allowed him to learn at his own pace, with no pressure to keep up with a school's schedule. Within weeks, Ethan's meltdowns decreased and his love for learning increased. His parents saw a huge improvement in his communication skills, as the one-to-one approach allowed them to model and practise language in a relaxed setting. The ability to tailor his education to his needs transformed Ethan's learning experience, giving him the space to grow both academically and, more importantly, emotionally. Homeschooling can be such a great fit for a neurodivergent child, allowing for flexibility and sensory-sensitive learning.

Is schooling from home isolating?

The single biggest reason parents give me for not wanting to do school from home is a fear of social isolation.

When well-meaning friends and family discovered we had chosen to school Chloé at home, they were concerned she would miss out on social skills and friendships. The school she was attending at the time told us they thought it was a huge mistake, because we were 'giving in to her' and would cause her to be more socially isolated than she already was.

It turns out they could not have been further from the truth. I distinctly remember the first morning Chloé woke up after we pulled her out of school. For the first time in years, she had no headache or stomach-ache, and she looked happy and relaxed – as if the weight of the world had been lifted from her. It is no exaggeration to say this happened literally *overnight*.

Chloé showed a keen interest in photography, so we bought her a camera. She loved art, so we ensured she had plenty of pencils, watercolours, oil paints and canvases. Despite her poor coordination, painful shyness and at times being selectively mute, she had dreams of being an actor and dancer, so we enrolled her in drama and dance classes. The first dance school promptly told me after Chloé's first class that she lacked coordination and skill, and we would be better investing our time and money in an alternative activity. So we did, going straight across the road to another dance school, where she bloomed because she was adored and nurtured. Just ten years later, she would be shortlisted as a dancer for the hugely successful kids TV show *Hi-5*.

While Chloé had always had horses and ridden, she started asking to join the local pony club and attend gymkhanas with her ponies. Before long, she was socialising and making *friends*. Little groups of girls at each of these places greeted her, got to know her and *liked* her because they had interests in common. Suddenly, without even trying, our little girl who had never had a friend at school, who had never fit in or socialised, had little groups of friends all over the place.

So, in fact, the very opposite of what everyone warned us about had happened. By pulling her out of a toxic environment where she was bullied and tormented and made to feel different and intentionally left out, she became happier, calmer and more relaxed. Suddenly she was able to just be Chloé. And by just being Chloé and having the time and energy to enjoy different activities, she was actively making friends with common interests. To them she wasn't the weird kid who stood out, she was a fellow ballerina, a fellow drama student, a fellow horserider. When she stopped trying, Chloé started making friends. Suddenly her life, and ours, was so much easier and happier. She wasn't just surviving, she was *thriving*.

Please do not think I am saying schooling from home is the only option. I know for many it is a luxury they can't afford, especially for families in which both parents have to work outside of the home, or for parents who simply cannot be home with their child all day. If this is your situation, my advice is to focus on finding the neuro-friendliest school that you can near you and working with them to ensure your child is accommodated in the ways they need.

Bullying

Nothing breaks my heart more than hearing a child is being bullied at school. Having seen it happen for years to my own girl, it triggers so much sadness in me to see it continuing despite every school loudly proclaiming to be anti-bullying. Kids can be so cruel, teenage girls particularly so. They seem to have an incredible knack for spotting even the smallest difference in others, and our neurodivergent kids are particularly susceptible to bullying, especially in mainstream schools. This could be attributed to the fact that neurotypical peers generally struggle to understand the way our kids interact and communicate, which can cause peer rejection or difficulties in establishing and keeping friendships. But, also, sometimes kids can be just plain mean, and our kid happens to be the chosen victim.

A note to Chloé:

I am so, SO sorry that for almost nine long years, we forced you kicking and screaming and crying into an environment where you felt so unsafe, terrified and alone that the trauma affected your mental health for years after, and still does to this very day.

I am so, SO sorry we didn't see you and didn't listen to you. Instead we listened to the so-called 'professionals',

the teachers who told us you were just being naughty,
you would grow out of it, we shouldn't let you get away
with it . . . who told us to just leave you at school and
not give in to your tears.

I am so, SO sorry we left you somewhere that you were
so afraid you hid in the toilets, and that the lasting
impact of school made you have a full-blown panic
attack on the first day you filmed Heartbreak High,
when you had to walk into a school and hear the bell.

At no other time would we knowingly send our child, crying and terrified, into an environment where they are being bullied or attacked, and drive off knowing they would be subjected to this for 6.5 hours a day. And yet for many of our kids, this is what school is like for them, day in, day out.

My *only* regret with pulling Chloé out of school is not doing it much, much earlier.

When we know better, we do better.

It was heartbreaking when one of my beautiful young autistic clients arrived in tears one morning because the group of girls who had been her best friends suddenly told her they didn't like her, she couldn't sit with them and they wanted nothing to do with her. What makes it even worse is when schools tell you the behaviour doesn't fit the definition of bullying, because it hasn't been ongoing or repeated. As far as I am concerned, one bullying incident is one too many. All children should feel safe at school, and especially our neuro-sparkly kids who are already putting so much effort in just to get to school each day. The effects of bullying can be horrendous on our kids' mental health, self-esteem and school attendance.

The different types of bullying include:

- cyberbullying: being bullied online or via phone calls, text or email, which can be so hard as it means even home is no longer a safe place
- physical bullying: being physically hurt, such as being kicked or hit, or having possessions stolen or damaged
- verbal bullying: being name-called, teased, yelled at.

The first step in dealing with bullying is to educate yourself and your child about the signs of bullying, so you can both identify it immediately. We need to open up lines of communication about bullying with our children so they know what it is and are able to tell you about it if it happens.

SIGNS OF BULLYING

- unexplained bruises, cuts, scratches
- missing or damaged items or clothing
- falling school grades
- refusing to talk about what is wrong
- not wanting to go to school
- trouble getting out of bed
- changes to sleeping or eating habits
- being 'sick', having headaches or stomach-aches
- being moody, teary, angry

Bullying at school stems from a variety of factors, including differences in behaviour, appearance or abilities, making neuro-divergent children particularly vulnerable. Kids who stand out due to their neurodivergence may be picked on because they don't conform to social norms, making them easy targets for peers who seek to assert dominance or control.

On the other hand, those who bully may be acting out due to their own insecurities, a need for attention or as a way to cope with their own experiences of being mistreated or marginalised. Sometimes bullies mimic behaviours they see at home or in the media, or they may not fully understand the impact of their actions. Understanding both sides of bullying – why it happens and why some kids resort to it – can help parents and educators develop strategies to promote empathy, create safer school environments and provide support for all children involved.

SIGNS OF CYBERBULLYING

- being secretive or protective of digital use
- being upset after using the internet or phone
- spending more or less time than usual on devices
- being anxious when away from devices for a period of time
- being nervous or anxious during or after using devices
- changes in mood, including becoming withdrawn, angry, upset, moody or teary
- not wanting to go to school
- changes to sleeping or eating habits

Sometimes identifying characters in television shows, movies or books who may be bullies can help your child recognise one. For example, Draco Malfoy is a bully to Harry Potter and his friends. Explain why people get bullied, and also why people sometimes bully.

Help your child to identify ways they can deal with bullies. The first step is to ignore them and not engage with them. Often bullies want to get a reaction and if they don't, they move on. Role-play what they could do – social stories (see pages 115–16) can be helpful with this, too. Remind your child that if they feel unsafe or upset, they can always go to someone for help. Work out together who the people are that they can approach, including their teacher.

If you suspect your child is being bullied at school, contact the school immediately. If they are being bullied online, the first step is to report this to the social media platforms, with the option of reporting it to the Australian Government's eSafety agency if the platforms don't remove the content (you'll find the details on page 286). Bullying needs to be taken seriously, as we are losing too many young people every single year to it.

If your child is experiencing school-related depression, anxiety, self-harm or suicidal ideation, relentless bullying and school refusal, I implore you to seek immediate help. It is far better to pull your child out of school than lose your child altogether. It is simply not enough for our kids to *be* at school. If they are not *happy* and *thriving* and feeling *safe* there, it is likely doing more harm than good. You'll find resources at the end of the book to contact if you have these concerns.

While it is imperative that the school deals with the bullies, I also believe many of our kids – neurodivergent and neurotypical alike – will feel safer and more supported at school with structured, safe activities to do at lunchtime, when they are most at risk of being targeted by bullies. When a child has no friends, or school feels like an unsafe space to be, there is nothing worse than having to wander aimlessly around a playground for an hour. Imagine as an adult that every day at work all your colleagues head off for lunch together, leaving you alone – or all sit chatting at a table, intentionally leaving you out and ignoring you. No one should be made to feel like this.

Examples of safer lunchtime activities include being allowed to sit in the library, or engaging in a club activity, such as chess or anime. If your school does not open the library at lunch or have lunchtime clubs, encourage them to start these options. Maybe you can even work with your child to set up their own club, which they can invite others to join. They are likely only one of many kids in the school feeling left out at lunchtime, and the best chance our kids have of making friends is to connect with others who have similar interests.

I was recently working with the most divine neurosparkly twelve-year-old girl named Amber, who was being relentlessly bullied every lunchtime by a group of girls. As soon as the lunch bell went, these girls would find Amber and follow her, taunting her. The girls would keep a low profile to avoid detection while absolutely destroying this gorgeous girl. I knew my beautiful client was the biggest bookworm and loved being in the library. In fact, Amber's dream job was to one day be a librarian. So I encouraged her mum to ask the school if Amber could volunteer in the library at lunchtime, helping the librarian put away books and tidy up. The school agreed, and the librarian was absolutely thrilled to have help. She even made Amber an official *volunteer* badge. Every time the other girls approached Amber, she would proudly say, 'Got to go! I'm late for my job!' And off she went to her safe place.

As well as providing a variety of safe spaces for kids to spend their lunchtime, schools should be proactively working towards ensuring all kids feel safe at school. Sometimes all it takes is a *volunteer* badge.

Sometimes our neurodivergent kids don't even realise they are being bullied, particularly when it is subtle. I can still remember over twenty years ago when Chloé was in her first

From Chloé 🦋

I often talk about the fact that I was bullied in school for being autistic; and I'm often met with responses of 'I would never bully someone for being autistic', or 'I don't hate autistic people', or 'no one would bully someone just because they're autistic.'

Correct.

Because people don't often know what autism actually is.

There have only been a few times in my life when I recall being outwardly bullied because of being 'autistic'. The rest of my life I was bullied for being 'weird'. I was punished for speaking strangely and using big words and moving strangely and not having friends and not catching onto jokes.

I was bullied because I didn't look people in the eye and I kept a small piece of fabric in my pocket to fiddle with and I didn't showcase emotions in my face unless I truly felt them.

I was scolded for questioning social normality and for saying the lights were too loud and for not fitting ideals.

People don't generally bully people for 'being autistic'. People don't hate 'autistic people' but like hell do they hate 'weird people', and those who are different from them.

'Autism' isn't the issue. An innate distaste for those who present differently from what you've been taught is correct, normal and standard . . . that's the issue.

year at school, and a large group of girls who had never been nice to her asked her to go and play. She naively chose to follow them, glad to suddenly have friends. They led her down to a back oval, away from the teachers, and proceeded to rip off her necklace while throwing her beloved soft toy, which she took to school every day, over the back fence into some bushes. They laughed at her while screaming in her face, 'Did you ever think we would want to be friends with *you*?' Sadly, only days later, they did the same thing again to her – our kids are often sweet and trusting, which makes them very easy targets and vulnerable to falling for the same tricks time and time again.

Transitioning to high school

Going to high school can be super exciting. It can also be downright terrifying.

While our neurodivergent kids often scrape their way through primary school, helped by the predictability of each day being roughly the same, having one teacher for all subjects, and receiving a lot of support due to their younger age, high school is frequently where things fall apart. High school is so different to primary school: different teachers for every subject, each with their own rules and expectations; moving from class to class, so choosing a new place to sit up to seven times a day; the expectation that you will know what you need for each subject and have the ability to navigate your way around a large campus. Add in the hormones of being a teenager (see chapter 7) and the extra challenges that neurodivergence brings, and you have the perfect storm.

You can do a lot in the final year of primary school to (better) prepare for a (hopefully) successful transition to high school. I say *better* and *hopefully* as sometimes, quite honestly, there is nothing we can do to make it positive for our kids. But for many kids these strategies will help.

Choose the right school

The most important part of transitioning to high school is choosing the right school. To start, see the section on choosing a neurodivergent-friendly school on pages 124–6 and apply the same search criteria to high school.

When choosing a high school there are also several specific factors to consider. First, look for a school with strong support systems, such as dedicated special education staff and access to counsellors who understand neurodivergence (and are neuro-affirming).

It's also important to assess the school's culture, seeking out environments that are inclusive, understanding and proactive in preventing bullying and fostering peer-support networks. Check if the school offers flexible learning options, such as alternative assessments or modified schedules, which can help accommodate sensory sensitivities, social anxiety or executive functioning challenges.

Additionally, consider the range of extracurricular activities and clubs, ensuring your child will have opportunities that align with their interests and strengths, which can be vital for building social skills and confidence. For example, some schools may be very sports focused but have limited arts programs, which will be no good for a child who despises sport and loves to perform.

Finally, visit the school to observe the classroom environments, ensuring they provide low sensory spaces or quiet areas where your child can retreat if feeling overwhelmed.

Preparation is key

Once you have chosen a school, prepare your child with extra orientation days so they can familiarise themselves with it as much as possible. In the lead-up to them starting, engage with the school in any way you can: attend school musicals, open days or sports days. The more your child sees the school, the more comfortable they are likely to be with it.

Get their uniform early so they can practise wearing it at home. If the woollen jumper is too itchy, have it lined inside with a soft fabric. Having a small piece of their favourite sensory fabric sewn inside the blazer pocket can be a great sensory support that no one else can see. Silky, invisible singlets or leggings can be helpful worn under the uniform to make it more comfortable.

Social stories (see pages 115–16) about school can be helpful, including information about each class and teacher, and a layout of the school.

Practise using the padlock for their locker. Tiny, complicated code locks can be a nightmare for neurodivergent kids who struggle with executive functioning and fine motor skills. If necessary, consider asking the school to allow your child to use an easier version.

In the few days before school starts, begin to go through the morning routine. Get up early, try on the uniform, do the walk or bus route.

Ask the school if your child can visit briefly before the first official day. Perhaps if there's a student-free day before school goes back, you and your child can visit, see their homeroom, meet their teacher and put some books in their locker. Seeing the school without all the other students may help your child feel more comfortable.

Laminate a simple one-page 'about me' for your child, which can include strengths, interests, challenges and strategies with a photo of them. Get them to help you with it if they can. Ensuring each of their teachers has this, as well as a copy for any substitute teachers, means in an instant a teacher can find out what they need to know about your child.

EXAMPLE: ALL ABOUT SARAH

- Things I am good at (strengths): art, writing, drama.
- Things that are difficult for me: maths and science.
- Things that help me to learn: clear instructions and kind, supportive words.
- Things I like: soft lights and quiet classrooms.
- Things I don't: loud noises, big crowds, noisy bright lights.
- Important contacts: my mum (1234 567 890) and my dad (1234 567 891).

Get organised

Organisation is an important part of high school, and often a real challenge for our kids. Practising how to read a timetable, learning the layout of the school and providing some simple visual schedules with prompts for before and after school can be helpful.

One of the best tips I have for this is colour-coordinating everything for visual consistency. Support your child to pick one colour per subject: for example, blue for Sport, green for English and red for Art. It is very important your child picks the colours themselves, as often a certain colour will naturally come to their mind when they think of a particular subject, which means the system will work even better for them. For me, outdoor education is obviously going to be green, but for someone else it may be another colour. Purchase a folder and/or zip binder for each subject that corresponds to the colour, then anything to do with that subject goes into that folder/binder. Apply the colour code to your child's timetable or daily schedule, which will help your child grab the correct items for the day. If they have textbooks or anything else for their subjects, cover them in that colour or at least pop a coloured sticker on them.

Use tools such as a shared online calendar or app to track assignments, test dates and appointments, which both helps your child stay organised and keeps you informed.

Maintain communication all round

Once your child is at school, try to foster a positive relationship with the school and particularly their primary or homeroom teacher. Start by establishing regular open lines of communication with teachers, counsellors and special education staff to ensure everyone is on the same page about your child's needs and progress. Encourage your child to self-advocate by teaching them to express their needs and challenges in a constructive way.

Set aside time for regular check-ins with your child to discuss their experiences and immediately address any concerns. Check in with the school and ask them to provide feedback, too. A few weeks into the school year, have a think about what is working and what isn't. Ask to meet with the school so you can have a mutual discussion about how the year is going and what you think may help.

Academic expectations

We all – whether neurosparkly or not – have things we are good at and things we aren't. Our different abilities shouldn't be judged against the same scale. This is why I despise standardised testing (actually, I despise *all* exams). While some of us are creative and incredible at drawing or writing, others excel at maths. Contrary to the popular stereotypes (thanks, *Rain Man*), neurodivergent people are not necessarily savants or academic geniuses; just like the general population, we display a range of different types of intelligence.

This may mean that your child just will not get certain school subjects, no matter how hard they try or how much work they put into them. There has to come a point where you say how important is it *really* that my child knows all their times tables by memory? I don't know about you, but I can think of nothing worse or more boring than practising my times tables over and over. I would much rather be creative and excel at the arts. I can still remember my primary-school teacher saying to me, 'You won't have a calculator on you wherever you go, so you need to know this stuff.' Me and my smartphone sure showed him!

When your child is struggling with compulsory subjects at school, it's important to approach the situation with empathy and practical support. Start by trying to identify the specific challenges they are facing, whether it's understanding the material, managing the workload or dealing with sensory issues in the classroom. Collaborate with their teachers to develop accommodations, where appropriate, such as receiving extended time on tests, alternative assignments or access to assistive technology that aligns with your child's learning style. Encourage your child by focusing on their strengths and reinforcing that everyone learns differently and has subjects they prefer over others. Additionally, consider supplementary resources such as tutoring or online tools that offer different approaches to the subject matter.

Sometimes, you also just have to accept that your child simply may not learn a particular subject and that, too, is okay. When her primary-school teacher was getting flustered that Chloé could not recite any times tables, and implying that she would not be able to go up to the next grade because of it, we had to assure her that it actually didn't matter. Even now, some twenty years later, she doesn't know them – and I cannot think of a single time she has ever needed to.

You can support your child to find their unique strengths in a schooling environment by paying close attention to what naturally interests them, or the activities where they show enthusiasm and aptitude. Communicate regularly with teachers to gain insight into your child's performance and interest across different areas, and identify potential talents that might not be immediately apparent. Encourage your child to participate in a variety of extracurricular activities and clubs where they can explore new interests in low-pressure settings.

It can also be helpful to ensure your child has plenty of downtime after school and on weekends, as well as encouraging them to continue doing the things they love outside of school, especially staying connected with peer groups based on similar interests. These groups can be amazing supports if they're finding the school transition challenging.

School refusal

While some neurodivergent kids absolutely thrive at school, loving the structure and routine, sadly, many don't. Traditional schooling just doesn't seem to work for those kids, no matter how much preparation or support is offered.

School refusal – when a young person becomes so anxious or distressed about going to school that they do everything they can to avoid it – can happen for a number of reasons, and is very common in neurodivergent kids. School refusal is not the same as 'wagging' school, because unlike wagging, it's not hidden from parents or caregivers. School refusal is often referred to as 'school can't', because these kids may either feel too overwhelmed or anxious about something at school to face it, or they just cannot bring themselves to leave the safety and comfort of home.

The first signs of school refusal can be kids feeling 'sick' on school mornings, hiding under their bedcovers, being unable to get out of bed or move, crying or pleading not to go to school or being up and down all night the night before (often due to anxiety about the next day). For some kids, the very thought of attending school can cause physical symptoms such as headaches, stomach-aches, vomiting, shaking or panic attacks. The signs and symptoms of school refusal or school anxiety may also be more subtle – showing generalised anxiety, having more meltdowns, or becoming agitated or angry.

I have worked with so many families who have undergone numerous medical tests with multiple doctors to see if there is an underlying cause of the physical symptoms their child is presenting with – only to find they are all arising from anxiety.

It surprises many people that you can get very real physical symptoms from mental health challenges.

School refusal is hard for your child, but it's also really stressful for you as the parent, particularly when it impacts your own day. It may affect your ability to hold down a job, which may have financial implications. It is difficult to know how much to push your child to go to school, and it is common to feel anger or frustration towards your child, as well as fear, worry and confusion. School is also compulsory for kids aged five or six until they're seventeen, so you may run into trouble if they don't attend enough days.

The first step to attempting to resolve school refusal is to try to work out why it's happening. Having discussions with your child, their teacher and even their therapists (if they see any) can be helpful in teasing out if there is a specific issue that needs addressing. For example, they may be having trouble making friends or being bullied, or they may be struggling with the schoolwork, the timetable or a particular teacher.

Often, however, school refusal is not triggered by a specific issue. Certainly in Chloé's case, and with many of the kids I see professionally, it's a combination of all of the above. But also, more generally, Chloé just wanted to stay home where she felt safe, comfortable and relaxed. When she was with her family and her animals, she was free to be herself. Of course, we later discovered the level of masking she needed to do all day every day would have been utterly exhausting.

Ultimately, and despite what anyone at school says, you need to focus on your child's mental health *more* than their school attendance. If your child is no longer here, their school grades will be irrelevant. Ensure your child is offered the appropriate support, and keep open communication with the school about why and when they are not attending. The school can adjust their workload, including sending home some work for them to complete if they are up to it. You could discuss attending only some classes or days, if this helps. Make an appointment with your GP, get some therapeutic support and ensure your child has access to mental health and crisis line phone numbers and websites (you'll find these resources at the end of the book).

If you're unsuccessful in working through school refusal, you may decide that your child needs an alternative pathway to learn, even if it is just for a period of time. Depending on their age, this may include leaving school altogether, pursuing alternative education or working, or taking up a schooling-from-home option (see pages 126–34).

Sometimes the answer can be surprisingly simple. A number of young people I work with have simply needed to reduce the hours or days they attend school, which has enabled them to continue successfully where they are. One young girl, Eloise, was fine in the mornings, but by the end of lunchtime every day she was having disruptive meltdowns that continued well into the night after she got home. The school was punishing her with detentions and suspensions, and her mum was being called almost every afternoon to pick her up – it was affecting everyone's mental health. Upon exploring this further, I found that not only did Eloise hate lunchtime – it was often the time she felt the most left out or obviously different – but she was also utterly exhausted after a few hours of school. When I simply suggested the school reduce Eloise's hours, so that she went home at lunchtime every day, everyone's life immediately changed for the better. There were no more meltdowns, detentions or suspensions, and everyone was much happier.

Another young teen I worked with, Quinn, was fine the first two days of the week, but by Wednesday it all fell apart. Thursday and Friday were absolute write-offs, with both days often being missed. Again, we discussed the possibility of Quinn just being exhausted, and worked with the school to lock Wednesday in as a home day. So she would break up the week with two days at school, one day home, then two days back at school, with the two-day weekend to finish it off. As soon as this new schedule was put in place, there were no more missed days. Intentionally keeping Quinn home for one day ultimately meant she was at school for an extra two. So simple!

The most important thing – as hard as it is – is to be kind, caring, compassionate and understanding to both your child and yourself. If it's this hard and frustrating for you, as an adult, it is likely far more so for them. But if you can remain strong through the time and effort it takes to understand their needs and find the schooling pathway that is the best fit for them (and works on a practical level for you), watching your child thrive will be such a sweet reward.

Q & A

Q: HOW DO YOU KNOW WHEN IT'S TIME TO CHANGE SCHOOLS?

A: Our kids spend over 30 hours a week for over ten years in school, so it's critical this environment is working for them. Ultimately, it doesn't matter what reputation, facilities or resources the school has – if it doesn't work for your child, they won't be happy and they won't learn.

It is important to note that changing schools is not an easy or fast fix, and it will definitely not cure every problem. I would recommend it as a last resort, once you've tried everything else (unless, of course, you encounter an issue so major that you need to leave immediately).

A few signs it may be time to change schools are:

- You have had meeting after meeting to discuss issues, and nothing is changing.
- They are not doing what they say they will to support your child.
- They are not listening to you and your concerns.
- They are not accommodating your child's specific needs (for example, they don't let your child have headphones or fidget toys, if needed).
- There is ongoing bullying that is not being addressed.
- Your child is always upset about going to school or when they come home from school.
- Lastly, but most importantly, what is your gut instinct about the school? Is your child happy? Are you happy?

If it's possible, changing schools at the start of the year, or at least the start of a term, can be easier on your child, as there will likely be other kids doing the same. Involve them in the process, such as visiting the new school beforehand or helping to choose their new school supplies to give them a sense of control. But this is not always possible or appropriate. Children are very adaptable and moving schools can actually help to build resilience in children by exposing them to new environments and challenges that foster adaptability and problem-solving skills. When a child navigates the complexities of a new school, such as making new friends, and adjusting to different teachers and unfamiliar routines, they develop a greater sense of confidence in their ability to handle change. These experiences can enhance their coping skills and flexibility, which are crucial for managing future transitions and overcoming obstacles.

Ultimately, you know your child best, and deep down you will know when it is the right time to change schools.

Q: HOW DO I KNOW IF SCHOOLING FROM HOME IS RIGHT FOR ME AND MY CHILD?

A: Sometimes you have no other option . . . like when our psychologist told me we might lose Chloé if we didn't pull her from school. These words still send a shiver down my spine as now I realise how right she was. We could have lost her. But if you are on the fence and weighing up options, there are a few questions to ask yourself.

- Do you have time? Schooling from home needs one parent or guardian around during the day, depending on your child's age. Of course this can be shared with family or friends, or by getting engaged in a homeschooling group where people often take it in turns.
- Can you afford not to work? Maybe you can work from home or work at different times, but it is something to think about if you are currently working. If you don't need to work but have always wanted to study, this is a great time to do it!
- Can you be around your kids all day every day with little to no time alone? Sure, we love our kids, but not everyone wants to be around them all the time.
- Do you have the resources to school from home? You don't need much but you will need a computer, reliable internet, a desk and a relatively quiet space.
- Do you have the capacity to school from home? If you struggled enormously at school or have mental health issues

that mean you struggle to get out of bed, it may not be an easy or appropriate thing to do. Having said that, if you decide on distance education, you will have the entire curriculum written out for you, and teachers to correct, assist and support you and your child along the journey.

Just like choosing the right school, ultimately it's about what is the best fit for your child – and for you.

Chapter 6

Mental wellbeing

Mental wellbeing is the cornerstone of healthy development, especially for neurodivergent kids, who may experience the world in unique and often challenging ways. Supporting their mental health goes beyond just managing stress and anxiety; while this is very important, it's also about creating environments where they feel understood, respected and safe to be themselves. This involves celebrating their strengths, providing emotional tools to navigate difficult moments and ensuring they have access to the right supports. By prioritising their mental wellbeing, we help them build resilience, foster self-confidence and thrive in their own authentic way.

As I've already mentioned, neurosparkly people are more likely than neurotypical folk to struggle with their mental wellbeing. I won't lie; some of the statistics are very confronting. For example, 38 per cent of Australian autistic people experience anxiety and depression, with neurotypical rates sitting at 26 per cent for anxiety and 15 per cent for depression. Shockingly, autistic women are thirteen times more likely than non-autistic women to die by suicide. People with ADHD commonly suffer from anxiety, depression, substance abuse or disordered eating, while at least half of people with Down syndrome will face a major mental health concern in their lifetime, including anxiety, obsessive-compulsive behaviours or depression.

That's what we're up against. By sharing these horrific statistics, I'm not trying to throw you into a pit of despair but to spur you into action. It's time to put on your best glitter (or whatever you need to truly shine), raise your pompoms and be your kid's biggest cheerleader and advocate.

How to support your child's mental wellbeing

Let's start with the basics. As I went through in chapter 4, it's so important to make your home a safe, neuro-affirming space where your child feels accepted and valued. This involves considering and accommodating their sensory sensitivities, providing structured, consistent routines where possible, and encouraging your child to engage in the activities and special interests they enjoy. Whether they have a fascination (or, let's be real, *obsession*) with a particular subject, a creative hobby, or a unique skill, nurturing these interests can boost their confidence and provide a sense of accomplishment. It does not matter if they are good or not – what matters is that you encourage them to do what they love.

Practise actively listening to your child's needs and experiences without judgement. Let them tell you about the gentoo penguin, who holds the title for the fastest swimming bird, reaching 36 kilometres per hour in order to evade predators such as leopard seals – regardless of whether you have already heard it 1500 times this week. Active listening helps build trust and strengthens the bond with your child, as well as letting them know that they and their interests are important to you.

Opening the lines of communication with your child is crucial for building trust and understanding, especially when it comes to discussing things that may be troubling them. Many neurodivergent kids struggle to express what's going on inside, particularly with emotional or sensory overwhelm. By creating a safe non-judgemental space where they feel heard, you empower them to share their experiences, including the things that might be hurting or confusing them. Encouraging honest conversations will help you better support them, and it reassures your child that their feelings and needs matter – no matter how difficult the subject.

One of my young clients, Sophia, was becoming increasingly withdrawn and refusing to go to school on Wednesdays, saying she had a tummy ache or a headache. Her mum couldn't understand why, as she was happy to go every other day. During an equine therapy session with Sophia, we began to unpack what was different about Wednesdays. We discovered the language teacher she had only on that day was very abrupt and loud, and made Sophia read aloud every single class. For an autistic child with dyslexia, this is a nightmare. Sophia struggled to relay this to her mum, because she knew her mum was so excited about Sophia learning this particular language, which is spoken in her mum's country of origin. We sat down and spoke to her mum, coming up with some strategies together, including Sophia being allowed to wear headphones in class and also not being asked to stand up in front of the class to read aloud.

Outside the home, work with educators to ensure your child receives the support they need in an inclusive educational environment (see chapter 5 for more on this). Advocate for accommodations that respect and encourage your child's neuro-divergent traits and promote their academic and social success, however you want to define those terms.

Everyday interactions can be helpful to support children to learn about identifying their emotions. Pointing out characters in movies or pictures in magazines can also be helpful to teach how emotions may be expressed. In equine therapy, I like to identify what the horse's emotions might be. For example, if a horse's ears are flat back and its teeth are bared, we talk about how this means it's angry. We then talk about what anger might look like in someone else, and ourselves.

Chloé uses the phrase 'eye sparkles', believing that *everyone* (not just those fortunate enough to be diagnosed autistic) has things that they are good at, or really interested in. Your child's eye sparkle is something that makes them happy, something they love, something they can't stop thinking about, something that will absorb them so completely that they ignore everything else in the world. If your child hasn't yet discovered their eye sparkle, they will.

As Chloé's parents, we chose to invest our time, energy and finances in supporting her to find her eye sparkles. Horse-riding lessons, ballet lessons, calisthenics, singing, pony club, painting and drawing, photography clubs and drama ... by spending time engaging in the activities she loved, she was able to develop her eye sparkles and find other people who shared the same common interests. She didn't have to try to make friends – they just eye sparkled alongside each other!

I recently had a parent and her neurodivergent teenager come to me seeking advice for how to find activities related to the teen's very unusual interest. I said to the teen, 'If you have this interest [obsession], surely others do, too, even if they are in another country,' and I suggested she set up her own group. This teen immediately got to work creating her own group. Facebook, Instagram, whatever social media platform your young person uses, get onto it. The world is a tiny place, and chances are if they are into something – even if it is the Cuban greater funnel-eared bat – others will be also. The group this teen set up has now attracted followers from all across the globe, where all of these people can get on and discuss their special interest with others. How cool is that?

From Chloé 🦋

Finding your child's 'eye sparkle' is so important. The world is a hard place, but when your child finds their people and learns just how magnificent their brain is *because* it's different, they'll understand that who they are is the best person they could ever possibly want to be.

Being supported in something that I loved gave me the opportunity to just be me. Riding with a group of 'cowboys', who didn't judge me for not brushing my hair (maybe because most of them didn't have hair) and only judged me on how I rode and loved my horse, gave me a time in my week to stop masking and just be Chloé, a fellow cowboy and horse lover.

Social stories

As I mentioned in chapter 4, many therapists and parents choose to use 'social stories' with their kids. Social stories are tools that may help neurodivergent people better understand situations, which I am all for. But it's so important to note that if we do use social stories, they *must* be neuro-affirming social stories.

Sadly, many social stories are designed to teach our kids to modify their behaviour to mirror neurotypical ways, tell our children how they should feel or teach them to *mask*. In other words, they are used to teach neurodivergent people how to act and look 'normal'.

Some common examples may be:

- 'I will make good choices! I will keep my voice, hands and feet quiet.'
- 'I will listen to my teacher, follow their rules and do exactly as they ask.' (*Eeeekkk*, this one is an extra big red flag – especially as a parent of a child who was sexually abused due to her being compliant and not being able to say no.)
- 'I will do my work quickly and quietly.'

Encouraging our children to act neurotypically by pretending and masking, and then rewarding them for this behaviour, is effectively saying that neurotypical people are superior and neurodivergent people are inferior, and we all have to play by the same rules.

How ridiculous. This is like making a social story for a kid in a wheelchair to show him how to get out of the wheelchair and walk. Or a social story to teach a deaf kid how to listen. 'Surely if we make pictures and stories about it, they will just *learn* how to do it.' I mean, how absurd and laughable. And utterly awful. It just would not happen . . . and yet here we are with similarly awful stories being pushed on neuro-divergent kids.

Neuro-affirming social stories understand the preferences, communication and interaction styles of neurodivergent people, and do not expect them to change their social interactions to suit their neurotypical peers. This means they will detail everything about a situation, including when it is happening, where it is happening and who will be there. They will include as much detail as possible, with specific photos if possible, because knowing decreases anxiety. The main goal of the social story should be about what the child can *expect* not what is *expected* of the child. School social stories could – and should – be for the whole class, and they should always encourage inclusion and embrace differences. You can check out some examples of neuro-affirming social stories on pages 115–16.

Social spaces

Sometimes stepping back and allowing children to grow and learn naturally, without formal guidance, can lead to improved wellbeing. Teenagers, in particular, need safe and welcoming places where they can relax, socialise and express themselves without judgement. Inclusive spaces allow neurodivergent teens to feel accepted and understood, reducing feelings of isolation and promoting a sense of belonging. Unlike structured therapeutic social-skills groups, these spaces allow teens to engage with their peers in a more organic and less pressured way. This, in turn, can lead to genuine friendships and improved social skills developed through real-life experiences.

Inclusive spaces also encourage self-expression and creativity. Whether through art, music, gaming or other activities, these environments allow neurodivergent teens to explore their interests and express their identities in a supportive setting.

This freedom of expression is crucial for emotional and psychological wellbeing, and is something our neurodivergent kids often miss out on. While therapy can be an important tool for supporting neurodivergent children, it is equally important to recognise when no therapy – or a break in therapy – might be the better option.

My brilliant autistic/ADHD friend Madeleine Jaine Lobsey told me about interviewing 200 autistic teens and asking them a simple question: 'What do you want?' They all said, 'a place to hang out'. While working for online platform The A List, Madeleine created social hubs for neurodivergent teens to 'be social your way' and just hang out, be themselves and connect in whatever way they want. She has amazing stories of the transformative experience it was for these teens to connect, including a teen who went from not speaking to having their first birthday party ever, at age fifteen, and inviting everyone from the hub. Seeing the magic created by neurodivergent connection inspired Madeleine to start her own social enterprise, Wondiverse, which now creates hang-out events for neurodivergent people of all ages.

By embracing your child's neurodivergence and surrounding them with neuro-affirming practices, you can support their development in a way that promotes their wellbeing.

Is therapy right for your child?

Due to the fact that Chloé was thirteen by the time she received a diagnosis of autism, she never had any early-years intervention or therapy. One of my first thoughts when she was diagnosed was such a deep sense of regret and loss that we had missed out on what I thought were important and crucial years of therapy. I remember feeling like such a bad parent, an utter failure. She did have a few sessions with the psychologist who diagnosed her, but this was more around explaining autism and supporting her transition to schooling from home.

Many assessing psychologists recommend therapy as the default solution once a neurodivergent child is diagnosed, framing it as the best or only way forward. While therapy can be incredibly beneficial to some, each child is unique and what works for one may not work for another. Neuro-sparkly kids often need a more holistic approach, which may include environmental adjustments, sensory supports or neuro-affirming strategies that embrace their strengths rather than focusing solely on remediation. Parents should feel empowered to explore a range of options, ensuring their child's needs and preferences guide the path chosen. I love this quote from Dutch author Alexander den Heijer: 'When a flower doesn't bloom, you fix the environment in which it grows, not the flower.'

When Chloé was first diagnosed, we didn't rush in to any therapy – we saw no need to 'fix' or 'change' her. Chloé has never had any specifically autism-related therapy, and we have never tried to seek help to 'overcome her differences'. As an adult, Chloé has chosen to work with a couple of amazing and trusted therapists who ensure her environment is best set up to suit her needs.

The right kind of therapy can certainly be of huge benefit to a neurodivergent child. But I also do not think all neurodivergent kids *automatically* need therapy. In my work, I often see neurodivergent children having several therapy sessions a week, going from speech therapy to occupational therapy, a psychologist and group therapy. To do this, they are often missing out on school, time to rest, time with friends and family, or time to pursue more enjoyable extracurricular activities. How utterly exhausting – not only for the child, but also for the parents – not to mention hugely expensive.

In my personal and professional opinion, it's better to carefully consider your child's specific needs rather than simply embark on all of the therapies recommended for neurodivergent children. If your child needs a lot of help with speech or conversations, then make speech therapy a priority. If they are having trouble with anxiety or depression, engage a psychologist or social worker. If they have extreme sensory sensitivities that you are unsure how to accommodate, seek out an occupational therapist.

The most important thing to confirm with any therapist for your neurodivergent child is that they embrace a neuro-affirming approach.

Neuro-affirming therapy

Therapists can be a wonderful addition and support to your team, but it's important to make sure they are neuro-affirming, which will mean their approach to supporting neurodivergent people emphasises acceptance, respect and empowerment. Neuro-affirming therapy is grounded in the belief that neurodivergent traits are not inherently problematic, but rather part of the rich diversity of human cognition. This approach is different to the traditional therapy approach, which has aimed to modify neurodivergent behaviours to fit neurotypical standards. A neuro-affirming approach means they respect and listen to the needs of neurodivergent people. They accept that all brains and people are unique, and that this diversity is what makes our community whole. They are strengths based, meaning that they see differences as normal and human, not as deficits needing to be fixed.

When looking for a therapist for your child who offers a neuro-affirming approach, you can start by asking how familiar they are with neurodiversity, and what their stance is on supporting neurodivergent individuals. Do they focus on celebrating strengths rather than fixing differences? Ask if they have experience working with neurodivergent clients and how they tailor therapy to individual needs. It's also important to enquire about their views on therapies such as Applied Behaviour Analysis, or ABA, which is controversial and undoubtedly harmful in many cases (see pages 168–71). A neuro-affirming therapist should prioritise building trust, respecting your child's autonomy and supporting their authentic self.

One of my young clients, Archer, who has ADHD, was struggling both academically and socially at school. His impulsivity led to outbursts in class, while his difficulty with focusing made it hard for him to keep up with his peers. His parents were concerned when they saw him becoming increasingly frustrated and isolated. We found a neuro-affirming occupational therapist (OT) who specialised in working with neurodivergent kids. From the start, the OT took the time to truly understand Archer's world. She didn't see his behaviour as needing to be fixed but instead as a natural expression of his unique brain. Rather than enforcing traditional, rigid methods, she tailored her approach to match Archer's energetic and creative nature. The OT used art therapy and hands-on activities that allowed Archer to express his emotions and ideas without feeling constrained by rules that didn't fit him. She also introduced mindfulness practices that were engaging and accessible for him, such as a short guided breathing exercise that he could do while moving or even playing with his toys.

In school, the OT worked with Archer's teachers to implement small manageable changes, such as flexible seating and more frequent breaks, which allowed him to better focus and engage. Over time, Archer began to thrive. He gained confidence as he realised his way of learning wasn't wrong – it was just different. His outbursts decreased, and he started building positive friendships with classmates, who appreciated his creativity. With the OT's support, Archer learned to embrace his ADHD as part of who he is, and his family noticed a profound shift in his sense of self-worth and capacity for expressing joy.

KEY PRINCIPLES OF NEURO-AFFIRMING THERAPY

- respecting individuality: recognising and valuing the unique ways in which neurodivergent individuals perceive and interact with the world
- fostering autonomy: encouraging self-advocacy and decision-making to empower neurodivergent individuals
- building on strengths: identifying and nurturing individual strengths and interests rather than focusing on deficits
- promoting acceptance: cultivating an environment in which neurodivergent people feel accepted and understood
- collaborative goal setting: working with the person and their family to set meaningful and realistic goals that align with their values, expectations, desires, hopes and dreams

If you decide therapy is right for your child, the benefits of a neuro-affirming approach include that it:

- Enhances self-esteem and confidence: neuro-affirming therapy can help neurodivergent children build self-esteem by validating their experiences and identity. When children feel accepted for who they are, they are more likely to develop a positive self-image and confidence in their own abilities without feeling the need to change.
- Reduces anxiety and stress: traditional therapies that aim to change core aspects of a child's neurodivergence can inadvertently increase anxiety and stress. Neuro-affirming therapy, on the other hand, focuses on creating a supportive environment that removes expectations to change, allowing the child to thrive at their own pace.
- Encourages authenticity: neurodivergent children will often mask or suppress their true selves in response to pressure to conform to neurotypical norms. Neuro-affirming therapy encourages children to be authentic, promoting mental and emotional wellbeing, by allowing them to express their true identity without fear of judgement or criticism.
- Builds stronger relationships: by fostering acceptance and understanding, neuro-affirming therapy helps strengthen relationships between neurodivergent children and their peers, families and educators. When children feel seen, understood and validated, they are more likely to engage positively with others.

You can even consider finding a neurodivergent therapist – there are many out there.

Stay away from ABA

If you are searching for the right therapist for your child, there are some red flags to look out for. Any type of ABA (Applied Behaviour Analysis) therapy, most commonly offered to autistic people, where the primary goal is to change their behaviour, is absolutely *not* neuro-affirming. It is based on the principle that neurodivergent behaviours are bad and focuses on modifying these behaviours through reinforcement techniques.

Often ABA therapy uses the method of withholding something from a child while we wait for their behaviour to change. Imagine for a moment if our partner did this to us, if they refused to acknowledge us simply because we didn't behave in the way they wanted us to. One of the primary criticisms of ABA is that it emphasises compliance over genuine understanding and communication. The therapy often focuses on making children perform behaviours that are deemed 'socially acceptable', rather than understanding their actions or the feeling behind the behaviours. This approach can lead to a superficial appearance of progress while neglecting the child's emotional and psychological needs. So, in many cases, people will report that ABA therapy is 'successful', in that they are seeing an improvement in behaviours they deem unacceptable. But this is simply suppressing the neurodivergent traits and encouraging masking, which can have a negative impact on mental health.

ABA therapy aims to reduce or eliminate behaviours that are considered undesirable, such as stimming, which, as I discussed in chapter 3, is a natural way for a neurodivergent person to regulate their sensory input, express themselves or cope with an environment. Having someone suppress these behaviours can lead to increased anxiety, stress and a sense of shame about themselves. ABA therapy is compliance based, so our children are taught that when someone – in this case a therapist – tells them to do something, they must comply regardless of how they feel or the impact on them. As I said earlier in this chapter about compliance-based social stories – and it's worth repeating – as someone whose child was the victim of sexual assault at the tender age of seven, this idea is very concerning to me.

The early implementations of ABA included practices that are now widely regarded as unethical, such as the use of punishments. The founder of ABA, generally considered to be Ole Ivar Lovaas, used electric shocks to stop autistic children from engaging in repetitive behaviours. In 1974, he was quoted as saying: 'You see, you start pretty much from scratch when you work with an autistic child. You have a person in the physical sense – they have hair, a nose and a mouth – but they are not people in the psychological sense. One way to look at the job of helping autistic kids is to see it as a matter of constructing a person. You have the raw materials, but you have to build the person.'

While *most* modern ABA practices have moved away from these extreme methods (and I say *most* because we still occasionally see abhorrent cases in the media), concerns about the ethical implications of behaviour modification remain. The focus on controlling and changing a child's behaviour can be seen as prioritising social norms over a child's wellbeing and autonomy. Many ABA therapists recommend up to *40 hours a week* of therapy, with parents encouraged to continue their methods outside of these therapy hours. So children are spending all these hours in therapy trying to change, when instead they could be playing, exploring their interests and being celebrated and encouraged to be who they are.

Any therapy that implies our children are broken and need to be fixed or changed in order to fit in is not okay. Essentially, it is teaching our children to mask the behaviours that make them look autistic. Studies on masking have shown autistic adults who mask are more prone to chronic mental health conditions, self-harm and suicidal ideation.

There is a strong correlation between undergoing ABA and experiencing PTSD. Many neurodivergent adults who underwent ABA therapy as children have told of feeling traumatised, manipulated and misunderstood. These personal accounts highlight the potential for long-term emotional and psychological harm, even if the therapy *appears* to achieve its immediate goals of behaviour modification.

There are still a number of ABA advocates who argue that ABA is not like that anymore. My response to this is perhaps

ABA AND GAY CONVERSION THERAPY

Both ABA and gay conversion therapy arise from the work of Ole Ivar Lovaas, and critics argue that both practices aim to make individuals conform to societal norms, rather than accepting and celebrating their inherent differences. This focus on compliance can lead to a person losing their sense of self.

By focusing on changing fundamental aspects of a person's identity, ABA and gay conversion therapy can lead to long-term emotional and psychological damage.

Moving towards acceptance and affirmation, whether in the context of neurodivergence or sexual orientation, is crucial for fostering a more inclusive and compassionate society.

once we have adults who have been through ABA saying it is respectful and helpful, then we can begin to have another discussion. But at this stage, I will be listening to the voices of those who have experienced it.

Alternatives to traditional therapy

There are some awesome alternatives to traditional therapy, including equine therapy, art therapy and music therapy. Think about what might work for your child and give it a go. Also, make sure you listen to them and to yourself. Your child is the best expert on themselves, and you are the next best. If they try something and don't like it, or don't connect with the therapist, don't waste your time, energy or money. Therapy is only worthwhile if it's actually helping your child.

Equine therapy

When Chloé was a little girl and really struggling with bullying at school and poor mental health, we noticed that the only time she was truly happy and relaxed was when she was around horses. Every Saturday morning we would drive a three-hour round trip to take her to a horseriding school, and as soon as we pulled in through the gates, she would relax, smile and become happy, calm and engaged.

Horses provided Chloé with a magnificent connection that she didn't have with any other person or animal. It was as if all her worries and anxieties disappeared when she was around these majestic animals. In fact, when Chloé was about ten, we decided to sell our inner-city home and move to a rural property, where we could have our own 'therapists' at our doorstep 24/7.

Chloé's magical connection with horses also planted a seed for me about equine therapy. A few years after completing my social work degree, I decided to go back and do postgrad study in equine therapy. From there, I opened a clinic specifically working with neurosparkly people, as I had seen firsthand the incredible life-changing impact horses could have on our kids.

Equine therapy is a psychological intervention that integrates horses into the therapeutic process. This therapeutic approach leverages the bond between humans and horses to promote physical, emotional and social development. For neurodivergent kids, equine therapy can be a joyful and engaging experience that also enhances various skills. We know that many autistic girls, in particular, are obsessed with horses, so it is a natural connection to make.

Horses are highly intuitive animals capable of responding to subtle cues from their handlers. Their sensitivity allows them to connect deeply with people, including those who are neurodivergent, and horses' non-judgemental and patient nature creates a safe and supportive environment in which children can thrive.

The major benefits of equine therapy for neurodivergent kids include:

- Improved sensory processing: horses provide a rich sensory experience that can help neurodivergent children more effectively integrate sensory input. The tactile sensation of grooming, and the sounds and smells of the environment can all contribute to better sensory processing. The repetitive motions of brushing, combined with the texture of the horse's coat, provide calming tactile input that can help soothe systems that are over or under sensitive. While the smells might feel overwhelming at first, particularly to children with strong sensory sensitivities, gradual and structured exposure during grooming can help desensitise a child in a safe and supportive environment. Therapists can introduce sensory experiences slowly, using grounding techniques such as deep breathing or wearing sensory-friendly clothing, helping the child engage without feeling overwhelmed. Over time, the sensory input from grooming – textures, smells and even the presence of a horse – can become more manageable, allowing the child to feel more in control and comfortable in their surroundings.

- Boost in self-esteem: the sense of accomplishment that comes from successfully caring for a horse, or overcoming fears or obstacles in working with horses, can lead to increased confidence and a more positive self-image, which is often lacking in neurodivergent children.
- Calming effects: a horse's gentle presence can help reduce anxiety and stress levels in neurodivergent kids, promoting emotional regulation and a sense of calm.
- Use of nonverbal cues: interacting with horses requires nonverbal communication, which can be beneficial particularly for neurodivergent children who may struggle with spoken communication. Learning to read the horse's body language and respond appropriately can enhance the child's ability to understand and use nonverbal cues, which can then translate to human communication.

Equine therapy offers a unique and beautiful approach to supporting neurodivergent children, providing physical, emotional and social benefits through the special bond between humans and horses.

Emma is a nine-year-old autistic girl who faced challenges with verbal communication, sensory processing and social interaction. When her parents brought her to see me, she was experiencing high levels of anxiety and finding new environments and activities so overwhelming that it was impacting on all aspects of her life, particularly school. In the first session I introduced Emma to a kind and gentle pony, Charlotte, and Emma initially observed Charlotte from a distance to help her feel comfortable. Over the next several weeks, I introduced Emma to grooming Charlotte, and eventually she had enough confidence to attach a lead rope and walk her around, first with me by her side, and eventually alone.

Being exposed to different textures and smells – including touching and brushing Charlotte – helped Emma begin to process sensory input more effectively. Successfully learning to lead Charlotte around the paddock boosted Emma's self-esteem, and gave her a sense of accomplishment and pride in her abilities. Emma's parents commented week by week at the positive transformation of their daughter – and all while Emma thought she was just coming to hang out with ponies.

Equine therapy can also be helpful to treat neurodivergent people with eating disorders. While traditional treatment focuses on food and body image, many eating disorders are triggered by unresolved emotional issues that need to be addressed in order to heal. Many people with eating disorders also have certain personality traits including perfectionism and rigidity – and around 70 per cent of those with eating disorders also experience at least one other mental health challenge, including depression, anxiety, OCD, PTSD or substance abuse.

Both neurodivergent people and those suffering eating disorders commonly struggle to emotionally connect with people or get too close, often for fear of abandonment. Many have also experienced trauma and have difficulty trusting others. Building a relationship with a horse in a safe environment can help them work through the feelings and process the fears that tend to come up in relationships. A horse can be the bridge for children to ease into communication when talking directly to a therapist can be too threatening, offering unique healing potential during the recovery process. Working with horses also allows traumatised kids to regain a sense of control and reclaim power over their lives.

Art therapy

Art therapy offers a creative and supportive way for neuro-divergent children to express themselves, often bypassing the challenges they may face with traditional verbal communication. Through drawing, painting or sculpting, children can explore their emotions, thoughts and experiences in a non-judgemental space that celebrates their individuality. Art therapy also helps develop fine motor skills, encourages sensory integration and provides a calming outlet for children who may feel overwhelmed. It fosters self-esteem by allowing children to create something that is uniquely theirs, while therapists can use the artwork as a tool to better understand and support the child's emotional needs and perspectives.

Music therapy

Music therapy provides an engaging way to support emotional, social and cognitive development. Through rhythm, melody and movement, music therapy taps into nonverbal forms of communication, allowing children to express themselves freely and connect with others in ways that feel natural. Music can help regulate emotions, reduce anxiety and improve focus, while also promoting sensory integration through the combination of sounds, touch and movement. Whether a child is playing instruments, singing or simply listening, music therapy meets them where they are, offering a joyful and neuro-affirming way to build confidence, communication skills and self-awareness.

Serious danger signs

While we are making progress every day to create a more neuro-affirming world for our kids, we still have a long way to go. This means that sometimes, despite all the love and support you provide, your child may still develop an eating disorder, anxiety or depression, substance abuse or suicidal ideation. We all need to be vigilant for any signs of these and immediately seek professional help if we find them.

Eating disorders

The most commonly recognised eating disorders are anorexia nervosa, bulimia nervosa and binge-eating disorder. Anorexia nervosa involves self-imposed extreme calorie restriction, which often results in dangerously low body weight and a distorted body image. Bulimia involves episodes of extreme binge eating followed by purging by inducing vomiting, excessive use of laxatives or excessive exercising to compensate for the calories consumed. Binge-eating disorder involves episodes of extreme binge eating without the purging part.

There is recent research to suggest a link between autism and anorexia. In fact, some studies show that 20 to 35 per cent of women with anorexia also meet the clinical diagnosis for autism.

This makes sense, given that controlling their eating can be a way of managing overwhelming feelings of anxiety. People with ADHD, meanwhile, are more prone to bulimia nervosa and binge-eating disorder. Neurodivergent – particularly autistic – people and those suffering eating disorders share a number of traits, including difficulties with emotional regulation as well as a strong adherence to routine.

ARFID (avoidant/restrictive food intake disorder) is categorised by eating a very limited variety of preferred foods. This can lead to those with ARFID being underweight and undernourished, because their persistent food restrictions means their nutritional needs are likely not being met. ARFID frequently co-occurs with autism, which again makes sense given how many autistic people eat restricted diets.

Eating disorders are extremely serious, with anorexia having the highest mortality rate of any mental illness, and autistic girls being disproportionately affected by it. While the exact reasons are not yet known, it may be that dieting and weight loss can give them some sense of power, control and self-worth – particularly when they are more vulnerable to being bullied and socially isolated by the 'mean girls', as well as often having social anxiety and sensory processing problems. Highly restrictive diets requiring routine and ritual can also naturally lead to eating less often and smaller amounts of foods.

Given the high mortality rates, if you believe your child has an eating disorder you absolutely *must* seek expert advice as soon as possible. But a word of warning: while autism and anorexia often go hand in hand, much of the treatment for anorexia is anything but autism friendly. Sensory needs are commonly not considered, and research suggests autistic people generally do not respond as well to traditional eating disorder treatment models, tending to have worse outcomes than non-autistic peers.

As such, it is imperative treatment takes a person-centred approach to accommodate autistic people's needs, such as sensory sensitivities. Autistic people experiencing eating disorders need access to a treatment plan that actively understands their worldview.

I have heard so many stories of 'professionals' who seemed to have no understanding of autism in the context of eating disorders. One family told me that when their daughter Amelia was seeking inpatient treatment for anorexia, the dietician was trying to make her eat foods she had been unable to eat since she was two years old. The dietician persisted in putting this particular food on her diet plan day after day, despite the young woman and her family explaining that it had always been off limits. The family tried to explain that the issue with this specific food was autism related, very common, and absolutely nothing to do with the anorexia. But the dietician proceeded to tell her family their daughter was manipulating them, and this was just another aspect of the eating disorder.

I have seen and heard of so many autistic girls who have rapidly got far worse when seeking traditional therapeutic supports for eating disorders, because their autism was being ignored. For a positive outcome there needs to be a focus on both the eating disorder *and* the autism – you simply cannot separate them. Even then, you will still need to keep an eye on the professionals, of course, to ensure they are treating the eating disorder, not the autism.

You are the expert on your child – more so than any professional, regardless of their qualifications. You are also your child's biggest advocate. Do not be afraid to speak up, especially when they cannot use their own voice to do so.

For us, what worked with Chloé was focusing *not* on the anorexia but instead on the consequences of not eating. For example, 'If you don't eat, you won't have the strength to ride your horse, which mean you won't be able to compete at pony club next month.' The alternative treatments such as art, music or equine-assisted psychotherapy, which I set out above, can be so valuable, too.

Neurodivergent children, in my experience, are often highly intelligent and insightful, so appealing to their intellect and common sense can be a valuable way of dealing with anorexia. One of my young clients, Arabella, who has battled anorexia for a number of years, loves dancing and is a promising ballerina. When I explained to her that severely restricting food intake and being underweight weakens bones, which can lead to osteoporosis and an increased likelihood of bone fractures and would forever impact her dancing, she listened. In fact, after our first session, her mum called me to say she had opened up more to me in our first hour than over a year of therapy with a psychiatrist and two 'eating disorder specialist' psychologists.

It is also important to note that neurodivergent kids frequently want to become vegetarian or even vegan. This often freaks parents out, as they think their child won't get enough nutrition or that it is another restrictive eating diet. But we know one of the common traits of autistic girls, in particular, is a strong bond with animals. And contrary to popular opinion, autistic girls often have far *more* empathy than others, which can often lead to them not wanting to eat their animal friends. As someone who went vegetarian as a child for this very reason, then became vegan with Chloé around eight years ago, my biggest tip here is to support the shift safely – try it with them, if you can – and educate them on the need to get all the appropriate nutrients from a wide variety of food groups. Ironically, for us, going vegan broke Chloé's long-held habit of only consuming white foods. She now eats a huge variety of foods from the rainbow and is far healthier than before.

POSSIBLE SIGNS OF AN EATING DISORDER

- weight loss, or weight gain or rapid fluctuations in between
- wearing baggy, oversized clothes (to hide weight loss) or layers (to stay warm)
- eliminating whole food groups
- making excuses to avoid mealtimes
- feeling cold
- fine downy hair on body
- dizziness or fainting
- missed periods in girls
- excessive use of laxatives
- food going missing or being hidden
- maintaining excessive, rigid exercise regimes regardless of weather/fatigue/illness/injury

Anxiety and depression

As I noted at the start of the chapter, anxiety and depression are significant concerns for neurodivergent people, including children and teenagers. These conditions are often exacerbated by challenges in social interactions, sensory sensitivities and rigid thinking patterns. These emotional struggles can manifest as heightened stress responses, mood swings or withdrawal from activities.

Understanding and addressing these issues through a neuro-affirming lens involves recognising the unique ways in which neurodivergent individuals experience and cope with their emotions. Providing supportive environments, implementing tailored coping strategies and seeking therapies that honour your child's neurodivergence can help mitigate the impact of anxiety and depression. Emphasising their strengths and fostering open, compassionate communication are crucial for helping them navigate these emotional challenges and improving their overall wellbeing.

Substance abuse

Neurodivergent young adults are more likely than neurotypical teens to develop substance use disorders, which can often be linked to their efforts to manage overwhelming emotions, social challenges or sensory sensitivities. Neurodivergent individuals might be more vulnerable to substance abuse as a coping mechanism if they struggle to find effective and supportive outlets for their stress and discomfort.

Addressing substance abuse requires a neuro-affirming approach that considers your child's unique needs and experiences. This involves providing tailored support, such as specialised counselling that respects their neurodivergence, builds on their strengths and offers coping strategies. Creating a safe, understanding environment that acknowledges their challenges and supports their wellbeing can help prevent substance abuse and promote healthier ways to manage their feelings and interactions.

Suicidal ideation

Neurodivergent children and teenagers are, again, more likely to have thoughts of suicide than their neurotypical peers. This can arise from the compounded stress of navigating a world that may not fully accommodate their needs, alongside struggles with social interactions, sensory overload and emotional regulation.

Early warning signs of suicidal ideation in neurodivergent children or teens can sometimes be subtle but should never be ignored. Some key signs to look out for include:

- Withdrawal and isolation: if a child suddenly pulls away from friends, family or activities they once enjoyed, this can indicate emotional distress. Social isolation is a common precursor to suicidal thoughts.
- Changes in mood: look for extreme or sudden shifts to persistent sadness, irritability or feelings of hopelessness.
- Verbal cues: pay close attention to statements such as 'I wish I wasn't here', 'I feel like a burden', 'things would be better without me', or talking about feeling worthless or trapped, even if these things are said in a casual-sounding way.
- Risk-taking behaviours: engaging in reckless actions, substance abuse or showing a lack of concern for personal safety can be signs of underlying emotional turmoil.
- Changes in eating or sleeping patterns: noticeable changes in appetite (eating more or less) or sleep (insomnia or excessive sleep or lying in bed) can signal mental health struggles.
- Decline in school performance: if a child's academic performance suddenly drops, they stop caring about their future, or they seem overly indifferent to things they once valued, this may be a sign of deeper emotional pain.
- Giving away belongings or saying goodbye: this can be a sign a child is preparing for an end and should be taken very seriously.

- Preoccupation with death: a child who talks or writes a lot about death, dying or suicide, or who frequently expresses thoughts about these topics, may be contemplating self-harm.
- Self-harm: engaging in behaviours such as cutting or burning is often a coping mechanism for emotional pain and a warning sign of potential suicidal ideation.

If you or anyone else in your child's life notices these signs, it's important to seek professional help.

Taking a neuro-affirming approach to the situation is crucial for your child's safety and wellbeing. This involves creating a supportive environment where they feel validated and understood, seeking therapy that respects their neurodiversity and employing coping strategies tailored to their unique needs. Open, empathetic communication and involving them in their own care plan can help mitigate feelings of hopelessness and foster resilience, ensuring they receive the comprehensive support they need to effectively navigate their mental health challenges.

Q: MY CHILD HATES GETTING DIRTY OR MUDDY. WOULD EQUINE THERAPY BE WRONG FOR THEM?

A: Recently one of my gorgeous neurosparkly girls, Olivia, came to see me with the most extreme sensory sensitivities. Her mum said she had been seeing a psychologist and psychiatrist for several years to address her OCD-type behaviours. She could not stand even a single bit of dirt, mud, hair or muddy water on her. Any of these would send her into meltdown, and she could focus on nothing else until she was clean again. Her mum was so concerned she was spending her life unable to interact with anything or anyone due to her extreme sensory needs, given that a single exposure to any of these things could ruin her whole day.

Over a period of weeks, Olivia began interacting with the ponies slowly – at first from a distance and then eventually touching their coats, brushing their manes and holding the grooming tools. All of this began to desensitise her, and Olivia was so focused on enjoying her time with the ponies that she was not even thinking about her own needs. Without talking about it, she began to happily lift their feet, picking the dried-up pony poo and dirt from their hooves and brushing dirt from their tails. I will never forget turning to see her mum watching on, tears streaming down her face, as she commented that equine therapy had done in weeks what a psychiatrist had not been able to do in years. To say equine therapy changed her life is an understatement.

Q: MY FIFTEEN-YEAR-OLD SON WHO HAS ADHD IS STRUGGLING WITH EXTREME PROCRASTINATION AND LACK OF MOTIVATION, ESPECIALLY WITH SCHOOLWORK. HOW CAN WE SUPPORT HIM IN OVERCOMING THESE CHALLENGES?

A: To address procrastination and lack of motivation in a teenager with ADHD, consider breaking tasks into smaller, more manageable steps and setting clear, achievable goals. Using visual aids such as checklists or timers can help him stay organised and track progress. Establishing a consistent routine and incorporating frequent short breaks can also improve focus and reduce feelings of overwhelm. Providing positive reinforcement and celebrating small successes can boost his motivation. Additionally, collaborating with a therapist who specialises in ADHD can offer tailored strategies and support to address underlying issues and develop effective coping mechanisms for managing tasks and enhancing motivation.

For myself, as an adult ADHDer with extreme procrastination challenges, I find lists and timers are great ways to motivate myself.

Chapter 7

A neurosparkly adolescence

Navigating puberty is a challenging time in the life of any child – and their parents. It is marked by numerous physical and emotional changes as well as mood fluctuations. (*Oohhhh* those mood fluctuations!)

For neurodivergent children, puberty and the hormonal shifts it brings can present unique obstacles and experiences, from heightened sensitivities and more extreme emotional fluctuations, to the complex social and communication challenges that may arise between teens and staying safe on social media. Understanding these challenges and providing the right support can help your child navigate this critical period.

You may start to see more or new behavioural and emotional changes during this time, and neurodivergence is often diagnosed during puberty due to these traits becoming more obvious. However, sometimes entirely standard adolescent behaviour can be incorrectly blamed on being neurodivergent. I often work with families who assume their child's particularly challenging behaviours stem from their neurodivergence. I can absolutely confirm, however, that puberty can be a challenge for *all* kids, not just those with a diagnosis. (There is a good reason why one of Australia's top adolescent psychologists wrote a book on raising adolescent girls and called it *Princess Bitchface Syndrome* – if you have parented a teenage girl, I'm sure you can relate!)

Navigating puberty with a neurodivergent child requires patience, understanding and a proactive approach. By equipping yourself with knowledge and strategies, some help if needed from professionals (and perhaps a few bottles of wine), you can support your child – and yourself – through this transformative period, helping them thrive now and setting them up for the future.

SARAH'S TOP THREE TIPS FOR SURVIVING PUBERTY

1. Support your teen's emotional wellbeing above all else.
2. Communicate openly and honestly with your teen.
3. Address sensory sensitivities in all areas of puberty, including clothing, personal care products, hygiene routines and managing menstruation.

(Oh, and my ADHD brain wants to add two more for good measure: lots of deodorant and a sense of humour!)

Communication

During adolescence and puberty, the relationship between parents and teens undergoes a profound transformation. Puberty brings a whirlwind of rapid changes – physical, emotional and cognitive – that can leave both parents and teens feeling unsteady. For neurodivergent kids, these changes can be even more challenging, making effective communication between parent and child essential. Clear and honest communication isn't always easy, especially when the topics are uncomfortable or when you fear the reaction you might get. But it's important to remember that your role as a parent is to guide your child through these challenging years, and open communication can serve as a much-needed anchor.

Build a foundation

When you communicate honestly with your neurodivergent child, you're building a foundation of trust and respect that will last a lifetime. Your child will learn that you will support them through anything. This will better equip them to handle the confusion and stress that often accompanies these years, when they are figuring out who they are and where they fit in the world.

Courageous communication also teaches your child that it's okay to talk about difficult things. When you model this behaviour, you show them that facing uncomfortable truths head-on is not only possible, but also healthy. This is a skill they will carry with them long after adolescence has passed.

It can be so hard to go from having a child who may have once eagerly shared every detail of their day with you or been your little shadow to a moody, sulky teenager who retreats into their room and speaks only in single words or not at all – if you are particularly lucky, you might just get a grunt.

But ultimately the goal of communication during adolescence isn't just to make it through these challenging years. It is to build a lasting and meaningful connection with your child, laying the foundation for a relationship that will continue to grow and evolve as they move into adulthood. Communication is the thread that binds your relationship with your teenager, helping them navigate the world with confidence, knowing there's a steady, loving hand to guide them.

If you can make it to the other side of puberty and adolescence (without killing each other in the process), you may just be lucky enough to have a young adult who becomes a lifelong best friend.

Be straightforward

It is crucial that when we talk to our neurodivergent children about puberty, we explain the changes that will occur in a straightforward manner that is appropriate for their age and ability to understand information. Puberty is challenging enough without our kids becoming confused by abstract concepts, or ambiguous or implied meanings. Our kids especially need to know that period blood is red and not blue, as it appears on some television commercials!

You might think this is a silly thing to state, but one of my young clients recently got her first period, and she was shocked to see the colour of the blood on her underpants was red. Years of seeing television commercials that showed period blood as blue had given her the wrong expectation, which made her first period more distressing than it needed to be. Many of our neurodivergent kids have a tendency to take things literally, so it's our job to ensure we are giving them the facts as clearly and directly as possible.

Difficulties with verbal communication can make it particularly challenging for neurodivergent teens to express discomfort or ask questions about puberty. They may struggle to understand what is happening to their bodies and how to manage it effectively. I have found that visual supports and social stories can be easy and concise ways to explain the changes in puberty and what to expect. This can demystify the process and provide reassurance. If you have an occupational therapist, they can help you with this, but there are plenty of free resources online, too.

A SOCIAL STORY: WASHING MY FACE

1. Getting ready
When it's time to wash my face, I will go to the bathroom and get ready.

2. Turn on the water
I will turn on the tap and let the water run until it's warm – not too hot and not too cold.

3. Wet my hands
I will put my hands under the water to get them wet.

4. Apply face soap
I will use a small amount of face soap and put it on my wet hands.

5. Wash my face
I will gently rub the soap on my face using my hands. I will make sure to wash my forehead, cheeks, nose and chin.

6. Rinse off the soap
I will rinse my face with water, making sure to wash off all the soap.

7. Dry my face
I will use a clean towel to gently pat my face dry.

8. All done!
I will use my towel to wipe away any soap or water from the bench, and put my face soap away and my towel in the laundry hamper.

Respect all perspectives

Respecting the perspectives of a neurosparkly child involves actively listening and valuing their unique way of experiencing the world. It means acknowledging their thoughts, feelings and preferences without judgement, even if they differ from what is typical or expected. Understanding and respecting their perspective fosters a supportive environment, where they feel seen and heard, which can significantly enhance their emotional well-being, as well as strengthen your relationship.

Clear communication is a two-way street. As much as you want to impart your wisdom, it's equally important to be open to what your child has to say. Your child's thoughts and opinions may evolve as they grow in ways that surprise or even challenge you. Listening to them without immediate judgement or interruption can be one of the most powerful tools you have. It shows your teenager that you value their perspective and that their voice matters – even when you don't agree with it.

Likewise, it's crucial that neurodivergent children learn to respect the perspectives of others. They often see the world in ways that differ from their peers, and they may struggle to understand neurotypical social cues, empathy or abstract thinking. Learning to navigate different viewpoints from their own will help them build meaningful relationships, advocate for themselves and feel respected in return. If parents model respect for their child's unique perspective, they can help their teen understand that everyone sees the world differently – and these differences can be a source of strength, not division.

One thing we have always done as parents is to encourage our children to argue their point even – no, *especially* – when we don't agree with it. We have had many family debates around the dinner table, over everything from politics to sexuality, religion and war. Sometimes this will end with one of the kids leaving the table in frustration. We give them some time and then ask them to return and finish their argument. We reiterate that just because we may disagree, it doesn't mean they are wrong, and they need to continue to fight for what they believe in. This has led to some awesome heated discussions, where minds have been challenged and ultimately changed on both sides.

Be present and responsive

There will be times during the teenage years when it feels like you are speaking different languages – when your words seem to bounce off walls and your best efforts are met with eye rolls, slammed doors and silence. These moments can be frustrating and heartbreaking, but they are all part of the process.

Patience is key. Sometimes the best thing you can do is simply be present, offering your teen the space to come to you when they are ready. When paired with gentle open-ended questions such as, 'How did that make you feel?' or 'How can I help you with this?', it lets them know that you are available if they need you.

We like to use fun questions to lighten the mood, such as, 'If your parent was your favourite superhero, what would they have done differently for you today?' This is an especially great way to acknowledge that your response to a situation wasn't the best, and it gives your kids an opportunity to let you know how they would have liked the response to go.

This openness is so important as your teen begins to face more complex and potentially risky situations. Whether it's dealing with peer pressure, experimenting with new behaviours or navigating the online world, your guidance is crucial. These are the conversations that can be the hardest to initiate but are the most necessary to have. By creating an environment in which your teen feels safe discussing anything with you, no matter how uncomfortable, you are helping them make informed, healthy choices.

As your teen grows, so, too, will their need for independence. This can lead to conflict as they push against boundaries you have set. But here, too, communication is key.

Having clear, respectful discussions about expectations, rules and consequences with neurodivergent kids involves using straightforward language and visual aids. This will help prevent misunderstandings and reduce the tension that often arises during these years. When your teen feels involved in these conversations, they're more likely to understand and respect the boundaries you are setting. Begin by clearly stating the expectations and rules, breaking them down into simple actionable steps. Use visual supports such as charts or pictures to reinforce these concepts. When discussing consequences ensure they are fair, consistent and directly related to their behaviour.

Approach these conversations with patience and openness, encouraging your child to ask questions and express their thoughts. By maintaining a respectful and supportive dialogue, you can help your child grasp expectations while fostering a positive and cooperative environment.

The need for sleep

You might notice that your teen is turning into a bit of a sleep champion – staying in bed longer in the mornings and dozing off at the oddest times during the day. This increased need for sleep isn't laziness. During puberty, your child will experience a whirlwind of changes that require a lot of energy. Their body is growing rapidly, their brain is rewiring and their hormones are in full swing, all of which take a toll on their stamina. Neurodivergent kids may experience intensified sleep difficulties, due to these hormonal challenges as well as increased sensory sensitivities. To keep up with these demands, your child will need more sleep, often around nine or ten hours a night. This extra shut-eye helps them process everything that's happening both physically and emotionally. It's not just about quantity, though – quality sleep is key. Deep sleep cycles are when the body does its most important repair work such as building muscles, strengthening bones and consolidating memories.

So, while it might seem like your teen is sleeping the day away, they're actually doing some heavy lifting behind the scenes, laying the foundation for their adult self. Given that our neurodivergent kids can struggle with sleep at the best of times, it's important to encourage good sleep habits. Adequate sleep is crucial for their physical health, emotional regulation and cognitive development. Establishing a consistent bedtime routine, creating a calming sleep environment and addressing any sensory needs can support better sleep patterns.

Recognising that sleep disturbances are common during this developmental stage, it's important to be patient and proactive in finding strategies that work for your child. Prioritising sleep helps manage the stresses of puberty and supports overall wellbeing, paving the way for healthier growth and adaptation during these pivotal years. Help your child create a bedtime routine that winds them down from the day, and try to be understanding when they're groggy (and grumpy!) in the mornings or need a little extra time to recharge. One thing

I always tell my clients is if you can book important things like therapy appointments later in the day, your child may benefit. Remember, this phase won't last forever, but while it does, your teen's growing body and mind will thank you for the extra zzzs.

Physical changes for girls

During puberty, girls experience significant physical changes as their bodies begin to mature. Breast development is usually one of the first signs, followed by the growth of body hair in areas like the underarms and pubic region. Girls can also start to gain weight, particularly around the hips and thighs, as their body shape changes. One of the most significant milestones is the start of menstruation, which marks the beginning of their reproductive cycle. For neurodivergent girls, these changes can feel confusing or overwhelming, especially if sensory sensitivities make certain aspects – such as wearing bras or dealing with menstruation – uncomfortable. Providing reassurance and clear age-appropriate information is key to helping them navigate this stage with confidence.

Menstruation

Menstruation is a natural part of life for girls, marking a significant and *very* exciting (yeah, right!) milestone in their development. My youngest daughter got her first period at the tender age of eleven. When she woke up on the second day of her period and she was *still* bleeding, she angrily said to me, 'Mum, I *still* have my period. I thought that was it yesterday?' I replied, 'No, baby, you'll have it for roughly a week every month for the next forty or so years.' I smiled, trying to sound excited and positive. She was utterly horrified and *disgusted*. Quietly, I agreed . . . being born a woman can feel *so* unfair sometimes. Anyway, I digress.

For neurodivergent girls, having a period can present additional challenges due to their unique sensory, emotional and communication needs. As parents, understanding these challenges and implementing supportive strategies can help them better navigate this phase.

Preparation

Begin discussions about menstruation early, ideally from the age of eight or nine, using simple and clear language. While the average age of the first period is around thirteen, it is estimated that around 12 per cent of girls will get their first period between the ages of eight and eleven. From when all of my girls have been young, I have made no secret about when I have had my period, and I have involved them in looking at different pads and tampons in the supermarket when I was shopping. Visual aids, including books, diagrams and videos, can be helpful to explain the process. Create social stories that outline what menstruation is, what to expect and how to manage it. This can help demystify the experience and reduce anxiety.

Something every parent should do before menstruation starts is to create a period kit your child can carry with them. I created one for each of my girls, including pads, period underwear, wet wipes, spare undies and a plastic nappy bag for disposal. This ensures no matter where your child is when their period arrives, they will be prepared.

Practise with these supplies before they actually get their period by introducing menstrual products (pads, tampons, period underwear) that your child can handle and try on, to build familiarity and get used to the feeling of them. This will be much easier to do before menstruation starts than after.

Open communication about all aspects of menstruation is key, as it will help teens express what they're feeling and find strategies to make their periods more manageable, ensuring they don't have to suffer in silence. Neurodivergent teens who struggle with communication may find it difficult to express discomfort or ask questions about menstruation. Encourage them to express their feelings and ask questions. Be direct and honest, and provide reassurance and validation.

Menstrual products

The experience of menstruation can be especially challenging for those with heightened sensory sensitivities. For a neurodivergent teen already sensitive to textures, touch and changes in their body, the physical sensations that accompany menstruation – including cramps, bloating, the bleeding itself, as well as the use of tampons or pads – can trigger intense discomfort and anxiety. The sound and feeling of a pad rustling with every movement, the new smell of blood, the pressure of a tampon or the unfamiliar feeling of wetness can all become a source of distraction or distress. Add to that having to dispose of sanitary products and missing out on activities they love, when it is already so hard to fit in, and this can be an extra difficult time for our teens.

It is crucial to choose the products that best suit your child. Experiment with different menstrual products to find those that are most comfortable. In recent years the market has been flooded (pardon the pun) with an incredible invention that has literally been life-changing for Chloé: period underwear. These look just like normal undies but have a special gusset made of moisture-wicking fabric that traps blood and prevents it from leaking on your clothes. As well as being more comfortable and less messy than using a pad or tampon, they are also a smarter choice ecologically and economically. Using period underwear means no trying to insert a tampon – which can be especially messy, painful and confusing for neurodivergent teens – or stick on a bulky, uncomfortable pad properly. There is also no need to dispose of bloody used rubbish, and no need to even see the blood, as the gusset is black.

Period undies come in all sorts of designs, colours and fabrics, so there is always something for everyone, and they feel just like normal undies. You can even get period bathers now, too, which are incredible. At the end of the day you simply rinse them in cold water – I keep a bucket in my laundry trough during period time that my girls know to drop their worn undies in, then a cold gentle wash and line dry, and you're all done. No more used pads left on the bathroom floor. I have to say, I was really hesitant to try them at first, as was Chloé. I just couldn't wrap my head around how they would work, but they do, and they are in my experience the single greatest thing you can get to help your neurodivergent teen with their periods.

If they do end up using pads or tampons that need disposing of, it can be helpful to have this set up in the bathroom. I keep a little period basket with a variety of pads and tampons and brown paper bags, plus a small bin with a lid to put the waste in. Believe me, the lid bit is super important, as it gives your teen some added privacy if they don't want others in the household to know they are menstruating.

Emotional regulation

The hormonal fluctuations during a period can amplify a teen's emotional responses, making an already difficult sensory experience even harder to manage. Parents can help by approaching this subject with empathy and understanding, offering practical support such as trying different period products, allowing extra time for self-care, and being patient as their child navigates these new and often overwhelming sensations.

The hormonal changes associated with menstruation can also exacerbate a neurodivergent young person's existing emotional and behavioural challenges. Increased anxiety, mood swings and difficulty with emotional regulation are more common. Supporting their emotional and behavioural needs by incorporating a consistent routine can help reduce anxiety and provide a sense of comfort and control.

This is a good time to introduce emotional regulation tools and techniques such as deep breathing, mindfulness meditation and yoga. There are plenty of great free YouTube videos available, including exercise for period relief. Having a toolkit of coping strategies can be beneficial during any emotional fluctuations (and let's face it, periods can be times of *enormous* emotional fluctuation).

If verbal communication is challenging, use alternative methods such as communication cards or feeling charts to help your teen express their needs and discomfort (though a slammed door is a pretty clear indication!). Having some social stories to show how to change and dispose of a pad or tampon are a great idea, too. You can keep one of these in their bathroom and a mini one in their toilet bag to access at school. If you have an occupational therapist, they can help with creating this, or there are plenty of great free resources online.

Other supports

If your child is really struggling with menstruation, consider involving neuro-affirming therapists who can tailor strategies to help them manage their emotions and behaviours (see more on therapists in chapter 6).

There are some great practical tips that can help, too, including keeping a menstrual calendar to track your teen's cycle. There are so many great free apps that can help with this. Once their cycle becomes more regular and predictable, trackers can be helpful to prepare accordingly.

Educate caregivers and teachers – let the school know, so they can offer support and have a plan in place during menstruation. I contacted the school when my girls first got their periods just so the teacher could quietly check in and ensure they were doing okay.

Periods can be a real physical pain, so experiment with sensory-friendly strategies to manage the discomfort, including heat pads for cramps, soft loose clothing and weighted blankets for pressure. My girls love the stick-on heat pads that can provide wearable longer-lasting heat. They also love the soft-toy heat packs they can snuggle while receiving the warmth.

Having suffered awful periods my whole life due to endometriosis, I was determined to make periods 'positive' in our household. When each of my girls got their period, I bought them a special gift and a beautiful book with a loving letter welcoming them to womanhood, plus we went out for dinner as a family and celebrated with a period cake (don't even ask!). My son was so confused as to what on earth a period party was. Come to think of it, so were my husband and girls. I wasn't sure, either, I just knew I wanted to convince them that periods are okay. And yes, my kids and their friends do refer to me as Kris Jenner (the Kardashian girls' mum) because I am 'so *extra*' when it comes to celebrating.

However, despite my efforts to make menstruation a wonderful experience (what was I even thinking?!), my darling first-born Chloé was not having it. Firstly, my little Peter Pan did *not* want to grow up, so she was never going to celebrate becoming a woman, no matter how much I attempted to put a positive spin on it. As is quite common with neurodivergent girls, she dreaded growing up for a number of reasons, including that she associated it with unwanted body changes, boobs, boys and babies . . . all big no-nos for her.

My best advice for menstruation is to focus on finding the right period products for your child and getting a discreet and consistent routine sorted – these things will be received far better than a period cake!

Breasts

Next to periods, one of the most significant milestones for a girl during puberty is buying her first bra. For neurodivergent girls, this can be particularly challenging due to sensory sensitivities, so finding a comfortable bra is crucial. Look for bras made from soft, breathable, natural fabrics such as cotton or bamboo, and avoid synthetic, lacy, scratchy bras with itchy seams or tags. Seamless bras or sports bras or crop tops are usually more comfortable as they minimise seams, stitching, and hooks and eyes. Choose underwire-free bras, as underwire can be uncomfortable and restrictive. Bras with wide padded straps can distribute weight more evenly and prevent digging into the shoulders. This is not as important for smaller teens, but it's a must for those with larger breasts.

Consider your child's activities when choosing a bra. For active teens, a good sports bra is important to minimise bounce and offer support and comfort during physical activities, and lightly padded bras can offer modesty and support particularly if your child is self-conscious about their nipples showing through their clothing and drawing attention to their expanding bust.

Try before you buy, as a properly fitted bra is crucial for support and comfort – particularly for our neurodivergent girls. If possible, make a special day of taking your teen to get measured, and try on several different bras to find the most comfortable option. In my experience, the cheaper chain stores have the softest, simplest and most comfortable first bras. The added bonus is they only cost a few dollars each, which is great considering your daughter can go from an A cup to a double D seemingly overnight, so each bra may not last long.

Physical changes for boys

Puberty is a time of significant physical changes for any boy, but the journey can be particularly complex for neurosparkly boys. As the hormones kick in and the changes start happening, you might find yourself wondering if you missed an instruction manual handed out at the parenting convention. Particularly if you are raising a boy without a man in the household, it can be really beneficial to have a male friend or therapist to talk through these particularly challenging parts of puberty.

As your teen's body stretches and changes, it's like it becomes a foreign territory, and every day brings a new sensation to grapple with. Watching your child navigate these changes can be challenging (and at times comical). You might find yourself laughing when you are told the shower feels 'too wet' today or when the laundry detergent suddenly smells 'funny'. Through it all, the key to parenting adolescent boys is to keep things light and supportive. Humour can be a great way to ease the tension.

Just as with girls, clear, consistent communication is crucial in helping neurodivergent boys understand and manage puberty. Using clear, simple language and incorporating visual aids and social stories can help explain the changes they can expect to occur.

Sensory sensitivities

Many neurodivergent boys experience heightened sensory sensitivities, which can make the physical changes of puberty more distressing. For boys who already experience the world more intensely, puberty can feel like being front row at the sensory circus, with all the lights, sounds and smells that come with it.

Suddenly their skin feels different – oilier, more prone to breakouts, more sensitive – and there is now hair growing in places they have never had it before. The usual clothes that were once comfortable are now too irritating to wear, and let's not even get started on the new smells. Opt for soft, breathable fabrics that are sensory friendly and less likely to stink like synthetic fabrics. Teenage boys – we love them, but *boy*, can they smell, so anything to minimise this is worth buying.

If your child has always been sensitive to strong scents, their changing smell may make them wrinkle their nose in disgust. It's as if their own body has turned against them, and the introduction of deodorant brings a whole new set of challenges. Finding the right scent, one that doesn't make them – or *you* – gag is an adventure in itself, often involving many trips to the store and a growing collection of barely used bottles. Try choosing unscented, gentle hygiene products to avoid sensory overwhelm.

One of the teenage boys I work with, Noah, really struggled with the overwhelming sensory sensitivities during puberty. His parents came to see me about certain clothing suddenly feeling uncomfortable and making him sweat more, which caused him anxiety and discomfort throughout the day. He found the smell of deodorant distressing and his facial hair growth overwhelming. The thought of using a razor and shaving cream was just too much for him to even think about. We worked on addressing each of these issues for Noah, including wearing looser clothing made of natural, breathable, moisture-wicking fabrics such as bamboo and cotton, having more frequent showers, and finding fragrance-free deodorants that he could tolerate. His parents also found a gentle electric razor that took away the distress of using a sharp blade and shaving cream, and he was much more open to this. Noah gradually became more comfortable managing the physical changes of puberty in a way that respected his sensory needs.

Changing voice

One day your child is chatting away in their usual boyish tone, and the next he's speaking in a symphony of squeaks, cracks and unexpected bass notes. Welcome to the magical and often amusing world of voice breaking – a rite of passage that signals your little boy is well on his way to becoming a young man.

During adolescence, as your son's vocal cords lengthen and thicken, his voice begins to drop in the most unpredictable ways. One moment he sounds like his old self, and the next he's channelling a baritone with the occasional high-pitched squeak thrown in for good measure. This roller-coaster of sound can be a source of pride and embarrassment – after all, who wouldn't be surprised when their voice suddenly decides to yodel in the middle of a sentence? Neurodivergent teenage boys can find their changing voice particularly unsettling, especially if they have sensory sensitivities or struggle with unexpected changes. The deeper tone and different vibration when speaking may feel unfamiliar or uncomfortable, leading to anxiety or even a reluctance to communicate.

This is your chance to offer a little reassurance and a lot of good-natured humour. Let your child know that what he's experiencing is completely normal, and something every guy goes through, even if it feels a bit awkward at times. And don't be surprised if he starts experimenting with his 'new' voice, trying out different pitches or laughing at the unexpected sounds he makes. It's all part of the journey. In the grand scheme of things, voice breaking is a small but significant step in your teen's growth. It is a reminder that he's changing, maturing and finding his own unique sound – both literally and figuratively. So, as you listen to the ups and downs of his vocal symphony, take a moment to appreciate this milestone, knowing that each crack and croak is just another note in the ever-evolving song of his adolescence.

Erections and wet dreams

As your boy's body undergoes transformations, he might experience new sensations and emotions that can be confusing, or even scary and alarming. Two common aspects of this developmental stage – erections and wet dreams – can be especially challenging to understand and discuss. For neurodivergent teens, heightened sensory sensitivities can make the physical sensations of an erection or the dampness of a wet dream feel more pronounced and distressing. They might struggle to understand what's happening to their bodies.

It is important to approach these topics with sensitivity and clarity. Begin by creating a safe, non-judgemental space, where your child feels comfortable discussing his concerns. Explain erections and wet dreams in simple, clear terms that are appropriate to his age and developmental level. Reassure him that these experiences are a natural part of puberty, and that all boys will experience similar things as they go through these changes. Addressing these topics can be particularly important for neurodivergent boys, who might have a heightened sense of embarrassment or confusion due to their already present fears about not fitting in with those around them.

Providing your child with practical advice, such as how to manage unexpected erections discreetly or what to do if he wakes up in a wet bed, can also help alleviate some anxieties for him. For example, it can be reassuring to let him know that if he wakes up with wet bedding, he can take his sheets off his bed and leave them in the laundry, and take an extra shower to freshen up. We made it clear to our boys that if they stripped their bed and left their sheets in the laundry, we'd just wash them and pop them back on the bed, no questions asked.

Emotional changes

Puberty is like watching a nature documentary about metamorphosis, only it's happening in your own home. Your once predictable, cute caterpillar of a child is now cocooning themself in their room, emerging occasionally to demand snacks and then retreating back into the depths of their evolving psyche. And just when you think you've figured out this new stage of butterfly, they fly off in a completely different direction – only to land in the biggest pile of dirty laundry that they've insisted on keeping on their floor, alongside filthy plates that have become petri dishes.

Puberty can feel terrifying – and it is, in all honesty, so much harder than the toddler years, which *no one* warns you about – but it can also be an exciting adventure as you accompany your child through their journey of adolescence and on to adulthood.

For neurodivergent teens, whose emotions can already be intense and overwhelming, puberty can feel like someone turned the dial up. One minute they're cracking a silly joke and the next minute they're on the verge of tears. It's enough to leave any parent feeling like they're navigating a minefield. A child with ADHD, for example, may experience heightened impulsivity or mood swings. Autistic adolescents may struggle more with the social and emotional aspects of puberty, such as understanding and managing crushes or navigating complex social situations, friendships and relationships.

Understanding your teen's unique emotional landscape is key. Neurodivergent teens might express their feelings differently or have difficulty recognising and labelling their emotions. They may not always know why they are upset – or even realise they are feeling something at all. Patience is your best friend here. When your teen seems overwhelmed or out of sorts, try to approach the situation with curiosity rather than frustration: 'I notice you are feeling a bit off today. Do you want to talk about what is going on?' A simple non-judgemental question like this can open the door to understanding, connection and conversation. Sometimes just being there without asking them anything can be even better.

Our neurodivergent kids may feel things more intensely or, conversely, they might seem less affected by what's going on around them. If your teen is prone to emotional outbursts, remember that these are often expressions of distress rather than defiance. Your calm, reassuring presence can (sometimes) be enough to de-escalate these moments. Validate their feelings by acknowledging them, whether they express confusion, frustration or anxiety about the changes they are experiencing. Neurodivergent or not, puberty can be *hard*. Especially for the parents!

EMOTIONAL REGULATION STRATEGIES

If your teen needs some inspiration for regulating their whirring emotions, you could suggest:

- watching their favourite TV show or listening to their favourite songs on repeat
- maintaining a predictable daily routine to help reduce anxiety
- using feelings charts, journaling or mindfulness apps to help identify and manage emotions
- creating sensory-friendly places in the home to retreat and decompress when overwhelmed

- regular exercise and movement, which can help manage stress and improve mood
- creative activities such as drawing, music or writing, which can serve as a healthy emotional release
- warm baths and facials or massages to promote relaxation and emotional balance
- using positive self-talk to build confidence and self-acceptance during challenging moments – and model this for them by practising it, too
- breaking tasks down into smaller, manageable steps.

There will be times when your teen will want you around, and times when they will want nothing to do with you (the latter seems more likely during puberty!). Communication doesn't always mean deep and meaningful heart-to-heart conversations. Often, it is more about the small things, such as sharing memes, or quietly leaving their favourite chocolate bar on their study desk or a special body wash in the shower to show them you care and are thinking about them.

As each of my kids have hit puberty and started struggling through the teen years, I have made an effort to do little targeted acts of service I knew they would appreciate. These small moments of connection build a foundation of trust, making it easier for your teen to turn to you when they are dealing with something bigger and need your advice or support. When they didn't want to talk, I would try a different approach such as sending text messages – even if they were in the next room – or leaving sticky notes with simple messages of encouragement, such as, 'I love you so much and I am so proud of you,' or 'For God's sake, clean up your room' (look, we all have our limits when it comes to staying positive!).

You don't have to navigate the challenging journey of puberty alone. This is the time therapy can be helpful – a good neuro-affirming occupational therapist, psychologist or social worker can offer tailored strategies to help your child manage their emotions and behaviours (and maybe even help you, too). It is also the time to reach out to other parents and friends – puberty is when you really need your village around you.

Social changes

Puberty introduces a whole new level of complexity to friend-ships, crushes and navigating the social world. These social changes, including an increased interest in peer relationships and social dynamics, seem to happen overnight and can be particularly hard to navigate. Trying to decode the mysteries of teenage communication is hard enough without also being neurodivergent.

Friendships

When we think about the teenage years, one of the first things that comes to mind is relationships – whether it's friendships, first crushes or the confusing in-between space where your teen is unsure how they feel. Social cues, unspoken rules and the ever-changing dynamics of teen social life – where people say one thing and mean another – can be overwhelming. It's common for neurodivergent teens to struggle to connect with their peers and feel left out of social activities. It can be so tough to watch on as a parent, but it's important to remember that it's okay for your teen's journey with friendships and relationships to look a little different from your own or that of other teens.

One of the best things you can do is to help your teen understand their own social style. Are they the kind of person who thrives with just one or two close friends, or do they enjoy being part of a larger group? Do they need a lot of alone time to recharge or are they energised by social interaction? Helping your teen identify their social preferences can make it easier for them to find friends who 'get' them and appreciate them for who they are.

You might also need to play the role of social translator from time to time. Neurodivergent teens can miss or misinterpret social cues, leading to confusion or hurt feelings. When this happens, your gentle guidance can help them make sense of what went wrong and how to handle similar situations in the future. If your teen has a hard time picking up on sarcasm, body language or the subtleties of conversation, offering clear, concrete examples can be really helpful. For instance, a friend may make a sarcastic joke that your child takes literally. Your child may be confused and hurt and unsure how to respond. You may need to step in and explain that the comment was meant to be humorous, not serious, and later explain how sarcasm can be tricky to understand, and how you can look for tone of voice or facial expressions to help interpret what was said. This kind of clarity can help your teen feel more confident in social situations.

It's also important to acknowledge that friendships might not always come easily, and that's perfectly normal. Some neurodivergent teens might prefer to spend time alone or engage in solitary activities, and that's not a problem. Encourage your teen to pursue their interests and passions, whether that is coding, drawing, gaming or something else entirely. Often friendships can form naturally when they meet others who share their interests, either online or in real life. These connections can be real and incredibly fulfilling, even if they don't look like the friendships of their neurotypical peers.

For so many of the young people I work with, it has been their cosplay conventions or online Dungeons & Dragons gaming groups where they have seen friendships – or even romantic relationships – blossom. As I mentioned in chapter 5, if your teen is struggling with friends at school, encourage them to set up their own social clubs at lunchtime to attract peers with similar interests.

One of my young autistic clients, Georgia, was really struggling at school. After coming out as queer, they were encountering some bullying and homophobia, which made them feel left out and lost. We spoke about how there would undoubtedly be so many other young teens at their school going through similar issues, who probably didn't feel 'as brave' to come out as Georgia had. So we spent some time coming up with an idea for a group called 'the safe place for queer students' at school. Georgia made posters to put up around the school encouraging others to come to the library at lunchtime. Imagine their surprise when a group of nervous teens arrived, thrilled to have some peer support and make a connection with others. We brainstormed what these young people could do to connect: painting, making friendship bracelets, Pride flags and 'zines' (mini magazines). Suddenly these young people had not only a safe place to hang out but also a connection with other students, which could turn into friendships.

Crushes, consent and sex

When talking to neurodivergent teenagers about sexual feelings, it's important to be clear, direct and compassionate. Role-playing or using social stories (see pages 115–16) can help them grasp these concepts in practical terms.

First crushes can be equal parts terrifying and exhilarating for any teen, but they come with so many extra layers of complexity for our neurodivergent kids. Your teen may struggle to recognise when someone is interested in them, or they might not know how to express their own feelings in a way that feels comfortable.

The first step in supporting your teen through this is to keep the lines of communication open. Let them know that it's okay to talk about their feelings, even if they are confusing or over-whelming. You might say something like, 'Crushes can be really intense, and it's totally normal to feel a lot of different things at once.' If your teen does appear to develop a crush, you can ask gentle prompting questions such as, 'What do you like about this person?' or 'How do you feel when you are around them?' This can help your teen explore their emotions in a safe, non-judgemental space.

This is also a good time to start discussing personal boundaries. Neurodivergent teens might need concrete explanations about what's appropriate in a romantic relationship and what isn't. Talk about the importance of respecting others' boundaries, and their own, and make sure they understand that it's okay to set limits that make them feel comfortable. It is so important your child understands that the concept of consent means that both people agree to what comes next. Consent must be given freely and enthusiastically – no one should feel pressured – and even if they say yes to something initially, they can still change their mind at any point. Emphasise that 'no' means 'no', but 'yes' can also change to 'no'. For example, you could say: 'Imagine you're on a date and the person wants to hold your hand. You can say yes if you're comfortable with that, but it's okay to say no if you don't feel like being touched right now.'

The issue of rejection is never easy to face. If your teen experiences a broken heart, it can feel like the end of the world. A parent's instinct is to try to fix it, but sometimes the best thing you can do is simply be there. Let them grieve, listen without judgement and remind them it's okay to feel sad and disappointed. You could explain rejection along these lines: 'If you ask someone to be your girlfriend or your boyfriend and they say no, it doesn't mean there is anything wrong with you. People say no for all kinds of reasons, and it's important to respect that. You might feel hurt or angry, but you must not try to force them to go out with you. This is a chance to focus on the people who do want to be close to you.' Be sure they understand that even if it feels difficult, rejection is a part of relationships, and it's never a reflection of their worth.

Talking to your teenager about sex is one of those parenting milestones that everyone dreads, but when your child is neurodivergent, it can feel like you're gearing up for a conversation that's equal parts awkward and complex. Vague metaphors about the birds and the bees are not going to cut it. You're going to have to be straightforward, factual and maybe a little bit creative.

Most kids have already picked up bits and pieces of information from the internet, TV, friends or school, but they are likely missing the full picture. You could trying breaking it down as: 'If you are thinking of having sex, both of you must very clearly say "yes" before anything happens. If you are not sure or feel uncomfortable, that is your body telling you to wait. You can say, "I am not ready right now," and it is okay to take your time. No one should ever make you feel bad for not wanting to have sex or changing your mind.' And yes, you might need to repeat these conversations over and over again, because if there is one thing most of our neurodivergent kids love, it is clarity and repetition! There are some great free online resources to help with explaining sex and consent that are specifically made to include everyone (see page 290).

Social support

Look around for social skills groups specifically for puberty-aged adolescents, developed and run by health professionals such as occupational therapists and psychologists, as these can be great ways to teach your teen about relationships. These professionals can also help with developing social scripts that your child can use to practise role-playing to help them feel more prepared for real-life scenarios.

One of the incredible groups I was heavily involved with for a number of years was a volunteer parent-run group for autistic teens. We had a hangout room each week that a different parent would volunteer to supervise, and it was open to any autistic teen and young adult to come and socialise – or not. We would get pizzas and play board games, and over time friendships – and even relationships – blossomed. If there is not something like this in your area, I can't encourage you enough to organise it yourself. It is a beautiful thing to be a part of.

Relationships are a learning experience for every teenager. Your neurodivergent teen might have a unique path, but with your support they can build connections that bring them joy and help them grow. All we want for our kids is someone who can love, accept and appreciate them exactly as they are – quirks and all.

HOW TO START A TEEN HANGOUT GROUP

- Identify interests: choose activities that align with the shared interests of the group, such as gaming, art or sports, to ensure engagement and enjoyment. (If you are starting this for your child you have the benefit of choosing this interest based on theirs.)
- Create a structured environment: establish a clear schedule and format for meetings to provide predictability and comfort. When we did ours, we would arrive at 6 pm for dinner at 7, then games from 8 and pick-up at 9. It helps for the teens (and parents) to know the order of events and when it will finish.
- Promote inclusivity: encourage open communication and respect among all members to create a welcoming and supportive atmosphere.
- Accommodate sensory needs: consider sensory preferences by selecting locations and activities that accommodate different needs, such as having a quiet space or sensory-friendly environment.
- Foster communication: use visual aids and social stories to help group members understand expectations and interactions.
- Seek feedback: ask for input from the group on what's working and what can be improved. As they may be too shy to speak up in front of others, you could leave a suggestions box in the space.
- Partner with professionals: collaborate with therapists who can offer guidance on creating a supportive group dynamic and addressing specific needs.
- Start small: begin with a manageable group size to help ease any initial anxiety, and gradually expand as comfort levels increase.

- Offer choices: provide options for different activities or roles within the group to cater to varying interests and comfort levels. For example, we always offered a selection of board games, computer games, and art and craft activities.
- Encourage other parents to volunteer: it is good to have a responsible adult or two floating in the background. Try to get a rotating roster of parents going to share the responsibility.

Social media

Social media provides unique challenges and opportunities for our neurodivergent kids, and we're the first generation of parents to be navigating these treacherous waters. Social media platforms such as Instagram, Snapchat, TikTok and Facebook (although my kids tell me only us oldies use Facebook now!) offer a range of experiences, from sharing photos and videos to participating in group chats. Each platform has its own audience, culture, language and expectations.

For neurosparkly teens who may struggle with social cues and sensory overload, these environments can be both stimulating and overwhelming. There can actually be many benefits to social media, including providing neurodivergent teens with opportunities to connect with others who share similar interests, which can foster a sense of belonging and reduce feelings of isolation. It can be great for self-expression, with platforms such as Instagram and TikTok allowing teens to express themselves creatively through photos, videos and other media. Social media can also be a valuable resource for learning about topics relevant to neurodivergence, including advocacy and support networks.

Neurodivergent teens may find it so much easier to talk to someone from behind a screen rather than face to face – and therein also lies the problem. I remember when Chloé was young and had first joined Facebook – probably around the age of fourteen – and she was friended by someone and started chatting to them nonstop. When I asked her how she knew them, she said she had met them in one of her horse groups. I asked her how she knew they were the fourteen-year-old girl they said they were. She looked at me as if I was not understanding a basic point and said, 'Umm, their profile pic is a fourteen-year-old girl, and they said they are in Year 8 at school.' I said, 'You do realise they could put a fake picture up and just pretend to be a fourteen-year-old girl in Year 8?' Chloé looked at me blankly and said, 'Why on earth would anyone lie about their age or who they were?' She just could not comprehend, no matter how much we discussed it, that someone would do this or what their motive would be. Her naivety and innocence made her a prime target for anyone wanting to take advantage of her.

It was really tricky to find the balance between her safety and her participation in these online groups that were so important to her. These groups contained her only friends, and she spoke to them daily online, yet she had never met or even seen them in the offline world. For some neurodivergent kids, these friendships may grow through online gaming. For others, like Chloé, it is horse groups or One Direction groups – your child will likely follow their special interests to find online communities.

If we remove their access to social media, or don't allow them to game online with people or chat to strangers in their special-interest groups, we could be taking away the only friends they know. We – or other adults – may not consider online strangers to be real friends, but I can assure you that these people can

From Chloé 🦋

Don't be afraid of social media. Maybe suggest that your kid use a pseudonym to start off, like I did.

When I was sixteen, I decided to start a blog because the story that I was being told wasn't the story I wanted to live. I was not going to let that story define me. I reached out to the world and told my story. I felt like I was screaming at the universe. Imagine my surprise when the universe shouted back – there were millions of other people like me, and my entire life changed. Now I realise just how important it is for voices like mine to be heard.

As for periods, sensory issues are incredibly difficult when you're autistic, and these issues can go up greatly when your period comes along. As a twelve-year-old, the changes were terrifying, and I spent my first few periods in an absolute meltdown, begging my mum for some sort of medicine that would make it stop.

As I got older, I learned how to better cope with the change, but it was still so uncomfortable. Period products are painful, the discomfort of cramps is often heightened in autistic individuals, and the overall experience is one that I still dread.

Period undies – as opposed to tampons, cups or pads – have been a lifesaver, as have pain-relief devices such as the Mira Pro. I have also learned how vital self-care is on my period days. I don't have to get up and be a superwoman; I'm allowed to take time out to binge my favourite films, snuggled up in my bed with a cup of chai.

become the closest friends our kids will ever make. When Chloé, by then in her late teens, first arranged to meet in person the girls she had befriended through her One Direction fan page, they attended a concert – then they went and got matching tattoos after. If that's not a real teen friendship, I don't know what is.

Obviously, keeping your kids safe has to be a top priority, and some of the ways you can do that are:

- checking their messages (I did this, with my kids' knowledge, until they were eighteen)
- having a rule that you must know their passwords
- talking about what is appropriate to share with someone they are talking to online
- asking them to come straight to you if someone says or does something that makes them uncomfortable
- listening in when your child is gaming with people they don't know
- changing privacy settings so location and full name are not shared.

A big concern for parents is how much screen time or social media is okay. This depends on a lot of factors that will vary from person to person. One thing to remember, though, is for those neurodivergent kids who are schooled from home or find it hard to make friends at school, their only interactions with peers may be online. Pay no attention to what the 'professionals' say about only allowing half an hour a day, or whatever the latest fad is – you know what your child needs better than anyone. Obviously it can't take over their whole life, and there need to be some rules and boundaries in place. Our rules included:

- completing schoolwork or chores before getting online
- jumping off an hour before bedtime and reading or listening to a book for 30 minutes before lights out

- no violent or highly sexualised games, which are likely to attract older peers.

Cyberbullying

As I discussed in chapter 5, cyberbullying is a very real and very serious challenge that comes from kids spending time online. Our neurodivergent kids are already a lot more vulnerable to online bullying due to their difficulties in interpreting social cues, as well as being generally a little different from their peers. When we were kids, bullying stopped when you got home. Now bullies can follow you wherever you go.

Understanding the potential dangers of sharing personal information online is crucial. Apps that show your location or photos may identify where you live, go to school or work, and can increase the risk for our vulnerable kids. The fast-paced, intense visual and aural environment of social media can be overwhelming and increase the risk of meltdowns or shutdowns that other kids may witness. Sarcastic jokes and nuanced social interactions can easily be misinterpreted, leading to misunderstandings. We all know how hard it is to get your point across in texts or online when you can't see faces or hear someone's tone, and this is amplified for neurodivergent kids.

My client Liam is a sixteen-year-old autistic boy who loves gaming more than anything. He joined an online gaming community to connect with others who shared his passion (obsession). However, as he became more active in the community, the other online gamers began mocking his communication style, lack of quick responses and inability to 'get the jokes', which soon led to exclusion and bullying.

Liam's self-confidence was affected, and he withdrew not only from gaming but also from school. He became visibly distressed and frustrated. We worked on strategies for handling online bullying, including blocking offenders and reporting abuse, but we also identified safer, more inclusive gaming communities for Liam to join. A number of parents in autism support groups were keen to get their gaming-mad teens connected with like-minded peers, so they reached out to each other and set up gaming groups exclusively for neurodivergent teens, which the parents monitored to ensure a safer, more inclusive gaming community.

Staying as safe as possible

Thankfully, we can implement strategies to encourage safe and positive social media use and minimise the harmful risks. These include:

- Educate yourself and your teen about the different social media platforms, discussing their features, benefits and potential risks.
- Encourage ongoing and open communication about their experiences online, asking questions such as: What platforms are they enjoying? Have they encountered any uncomfortable or confusing situations? How do they feel after spending time on social media?
- Establish clear guidelines for social media use, which might include time limits or accessing social media at specific times to prevent it from interfering with other activities.
- Discuss what types of content are appropriate to post, follow and view. For us, it was imperative our child battling an eating disorder did not follow 'thinspo' accounts (yes, sadly these are a thing, and they're very popular, particularly with our vulnerable teen girls).

- Follow and connect with supportive and like-minded individuals and groups. We encouraged Chloé to follow body positivity accounts. (On that front, check out the incredible documentary *Embrace Kids* . . . you can thank me later.)
- Help your teen set up and regularly review their privacy settings to control who can see their posts and contact them.
- Use parental controls, if necessary, to monitor their social media activity and keep them safe, especially in the beginning (you may be amazed to know that social media sites allow easy access to explicit pornography and violence). You can gradually increase your teen's independence as they demonstrate responsible use.
- Participate in positive online communities, particularly those with neurodivergent role models, advocacy groups or interest-based clubs.
- Help your teen develop resilience and coping skills to handle negative experiences online. Teach them how to block someone, report someone behaving inappropriately or unfollow an account. Role-play different scenarios to practise responses to cyberbullying or other uncomfortable situations.
- Encourage a healthy balance between online and offline activities. Support your teen to pursue hobbies, sports, interests and social events that don't always involve screens. This can reduce the risk of becoming overly dependent on social media for social interactions.

Navigating social media is a complex task for anyone, even more so for our neurodivergent teens. But with the right support and strategies, it can also be a positive and enriching experience, encouraging friendships and interests that just wouldn't happen offline. By educating, setting boundaries, monitoring and encouraging positive interactions, parents can help their kids thrive in the digital world. There is so much to fear with our kids being online and interacting with strangers, but there are more incredible benefits that can happen as a result – especially those online strangers becoming real-life friends.

SARAH'S TOP THREE TIPS FOR SURVIVING SOCIAL MEDIA

1. Social media can be great – allow your child to make friends there.
2. It is your job to protect your child on social media, so keep those lines of communication open.
3. Set realistic time limits and boundaries, but allow yourself to be flexible.

Q: MY FOURTEEN-YEAR-OLD DAUGHTER WITH ADHD HAS RECENTLY STARTED USING INSTAGRAM AND TIKTOK. SHE SPENDS A LOT OF TIME ON THESE PLATFORMS, AND I AM WORRIED ABOUT NEGATIVE INFLUENCES AND CYBERBULLYING. HOW CAN I ENSURE SHE USES SOCIAL MEDIA SAFELY AND RESPONSIBLY?

A: Navigating social media use with neurodivergent teens can be particularly challenging, but with the right strategies, you can help your daughter have a positive and safe experience. First, open up a conversation with her about how she's using these platforms. Ask her what she enjoys about them, who she follows, and if she's ever encountered anything that made her uncomfortable. The primary goal here is to try to understand her experience but not make her feel like she's being interrogated.

You also need to set clear guidelines. In my opinion, fourteen is too young to have free rein over the internet, especially with these social media platforms. Openly discuss what kinds of content are appropriate to post and view, talk about privacy settings and adjust them so only approved followers can see her content. Encourage her to be selective about whom she accepts as followers, and to avoid sharing any personal information such as her location or school.

You can (and should for a fourteen-year-old) implement safety measures such as setting screen-time limits and using parental control apps to monitor activity. Educate her on how to recognise red flags such as inappropriate messages or photos, cyberbullying, or someone pressuring her to share more than she is comfortable with. Ensure she knows how to block and report users, and assure her she can come to you with anything if it doesn't feel right. Chances are, whether you like it or not, your daughter is going to be accessing social media. By maintaining an open dialogue and setting clear boundaries, you can help your daughter navigate social media in a way that is safe, responsible and enjoyable.

Q: MY AUTISTIC TEEN STRUGGLES WITH INTENSE ANXIETY DURING SOCIAL INTERACTIONS AND OFTEN AVOIDS PARTICIPATING IN GROUP ACTIVITIES. WHAT STRATEGIES CAN I USE TO HELP HIM FEEL MORE COMFORTABLE AND ENGAGE WITH HIS PEERS?

A: Helping your son manage social anxiety and engage more comfortably with his peers involves a combination of gradual exposure, supportive strategies and building confidence.

Start by identifying low-pressure social situations where he feels safer and more in control. Encourage him to join small interest-based groups where he can connect with others who share his hobbies or passions. These do not need to be with people his own age, either – if he loves photography, you might find a local photography group full of sixty-year-old women who are likely to embrace him and be thrilled to be teaching a young teen their skills. Use social stories or role-playing to practise common social scenarios and develop coping strategies. It's also beneficial to work with a therapist – if he has one – who can provide tailored support and anxiety-management techniques. Celebrate his efforts and progress, no matter how small, to reinforce positive experiences and gradually build his confidence in social settings.

Q: MY SIXTEEN-YEAR-OLD DAUGHTER HAS BEEN EXPERIENCING SIGNIFICANT MOOD SWINGS AND IRRITABILITY DURING PUBERTY. HOW CAN I SUPPORT HER IN MANAGING THESE EMOTIONAL CHANGES AND MAINTAIN A POSITIVE RELATIONSHIP WITH HER?

A: Firstly, you will need prayers, patience and prosecco to get through this! Supporting your neurodivergent daughter through mood swings and irritability during puberty also involves a combination of empathy, routine and effective communication. Start by creating a stable and predictable environment that helps her feel secure. Although it can be hard, try not to react to her emotional outbursts, which will often be directed at you. Right now, she needs calm and stability, not someone who will react in the same way she is. Encourage open dialogue about her emotions and validate her feelings without judgement. We all know puberty can be really hard, especially for teenage girls. Establish regular check-ins with her – these can be best done informally on a coffee date or a trip to the nail salon together. Identify what she loves to do, and make time to do these activities together when you can. Provide coping strategies such as mindfulness exercises or sensory tools to help manage emotional fluctuations.

I love spoiling my teens with little gifts that I know will help them through tough times. I recently bought my youngest daughter the most beautiful mindfulness colouring book and journal, along with a set of exquisite-quality textas, and she loved them. It can be fun to just purchase little gifts for no reason and simply leave them on their bed. Now, more than ever, they need to know they are loved, and you are thinking of them, even – no, *especially* – when they are at their most unlovable. Additionally, consider involving mental health professionals who specialise in neurodivergent adolescents to offer tailored support. By maintaining patience, understanding and open communication at all times, you can help her navigate these changes.

Chapter 8

Adulting

Adulting. This is how it goes:

You get your driver's licence. Tick.

You get a part-time job. Or two. Or three. Tick.

You finish high school. Tick.

You move into a share house with your friends. Tick.

You get a job, or go to university and then get a job. Tick.

You do some overseas travel. Tick.

You get married. Tick.

You move in with your spouse. Tick.

You get a dog. And maybe even a cat. Tick.

You buy a house. Tick.

You have a kid. Then maybe some more kids. Tick.

And you live happily ever . . .

Becoming an adult is *supposed* to look something like this, give or take the order of how it happens. But, while transitioning to adulthood is a pivotal stage for everyone, for our neurodivergent kids, this journey can come with unique challenges and opportunities. This means it won't always look like the list above – sometimes not at all – and that's okay.

As neurosparkly children grow and transition into adulthood, their needs and required support may evolve. But this phase also requires adjustments for us parents, both in what we expect from our kids and how we engage with them. Our job is to foster independence and confidence and to support them to build a fulfilling adult life – whatever that looks like for them. But if we believe what we are told by society, everything we do up until they are about eighteen is just getting them ready to push them from the nest. Our job is to train them up to not need us anymore (sob).

Typically this transition from childhood to adulthood is marked by changes in education, employment, social relationships and living arrangements. As parents we play a crucial role in navigating these changes and ensuring our children are equipped to handle this new life stage.

Encouraging independence

Most parents would consider that their child's journey to independence starts with encouraging them to participate in daily tasks such as cooking, cleaning or managing money, all of which are preparing them to move out of home. But while other parents I knew were practically packing their kids' bags and pushing them out the door, I was happily holding onto mine for dear life – and this was before I even knew anything about neurodivergence.

I've always absolutely loved having my kids at home. I am still happiest when I have my whole family there with me. There was no way at the age of eighteen that Chloé was ready or willing to move out of home – and there was no way in heck I was ready for her to, either. She had not even begun to learn about working, paying bills, washing dishes or clothes, or meal prepping and cooking. In fact, at that time I could not imagine her ever moving out, let alone getting married.

Our neurodivergent kids may mature a lot later than their peers, and that is okay. I often talk with parents about what an incredible difference even twelve months can make in our kids' abilities. I was consistently blown away at what our girl could do from one year to the next, and even though it may have been years behind a lot of her neurotypical peers, eventually she would catch up.

Even when Chloé turned 21, we were still so sure our girl would not be living independently, we had begun to make plans to build a second smaller house on our property, so we could always live close by and support her in any way that she needed. As I'll discuss below, I couldn't have been more wrong (although thankfully she is still only a couple of minutes down the road).

Encouraging independence in your neurodivergent child as they transition into adulthood is a journey that requires patience, understanding and a deep respect for their unique strengths and challenges. It's natural for us to want to protect and guide our children, especially when the world often feels unkind or unprepared for their differences. However, independence is a crucial part of their growth, and fostering it can empower them to navigate adulthood with confidence.

Practical skills

It's essential to recognise and understand that independence won't look the same for every neurodivergent young adult. For your child, independence might mean mastering *some* daily living skills, managing their time or learning to advocate for themselves in various settings. It could also mean knowing when to ask for help and understanding their own needs and boundaries. The goal is to help them build a life that is *fulfilling and aligned with their values*, even if that life doesn't fit the conventional mould.

Encouraging independence also involves teaching practical skills in a way that is accessible and meaningful to your child. Break tasks down into smaller, manageable steps and celebrate each milestone they achieve no matter how small. Whether it's learning to prepare a very simple meal or even a snack, manage a budget or use public transport, each new skill they acquire is one step towards greater autonomy. It's so important to be patient and recognise that progress might come in small bursts followed by periods of sitting still, and that's okay. What matters is the overall trajectory towards greater self-sufficiency, whatever that looks like to them.

Chloé's path to independence was a slow build over several years. It started with baby steps, such as going into the supermarket and buying groceries alone, or dropping her off to a concert but sitting in the carpark, phone in hand, so we could respond immediately if she needed us. We built up to Chloé attending concerts without us in Melbourne, then interstate, and eventually going overseas alone.

One of my young autistic clients, Jamie, was navigating the transition to adulthood and struggling with everyday life skills, such as budgeting and time management. Traditional approaches weren't clicking for him, so we worked together to break tasks down into smaller, more manageable steps and used visual aids such as colour-coded schedules and apps for reminders. Jamie thrived on the clear routines and found his rhythm by creating a structured daily plan that accommodated his sensory needs. Over time, Jamie gained confidence in handling his responsibilities and discovered he had strengths in organisation and problem-solving – helping him feel more independent and capable as he navigated the complexities of adult life.

Another one of my young adult clients, Eve, was wanting some independence but was not ready to live alone. Her aging parents, who had been considering downsizing for some time, decided to sell their large spacious home and invest in two smaller units side by side – one for them and one for Eve. It gave Eve the independence she craved but meant she was right next to her parents if she needed anything. While this is not something everyone can – or wants to – do, for this family it was an absolutely perfect solution.

Emotional support and growth

Another key aspect of fostering independence is supporting your child to understand and advocate for their needs. This might involve helping them recognise their sensory triggers, learning how to communicate their preferences in social situations or developing strategies to manage stress and anxiety. As they begin to take more control over their life, they'll need to be equipped with the tools to navigate the world in a way that honours and works for their neurodivergent identity. After being with them for every step of the way in childhood, you'll understand their needs so well, and it will just be a matter of helping them figure out how to express those when you're not around.

Supporting your child's emotional growth and fostering independence as they transition to adulthood involves recognising and validating their unique needs while providing opportunities for self-discovery and responsibility. Encourage open conversations about their feelings and aspirations, and support them in setting and pursuing personal goals. Provide structured environments and practical tools that align with their strengths, such as visual schedules or organisational aids. Allow them to make decisions and learn from experiences, offering guidance and reassurance as needed.

Additionally, it's important to acknowledge and address the emotional aspects of the transition. Both you and your child may feel a mix of excitement and fear as they become more independent and less reliant on you. Open communication is essential: talk about their hopes and dreams, as well as their concerns and fears, and share yours as well. Reassure them that it's okay to feel uncertain, and that independence doesn't mean you are no longer there to support them or that they have to do everything alone.

Build a support network of people who can be a safety net for your child while they explore their independence. The first time we put Chloé on a plane to Sydney from Melbourne to see One Direction in concert (of course!), we contacted our friends and work colleagues in Sydney, asking them to be on standby if she needed anything urgently. Knowing she had people ready to jump in, if needed, meant we could sleep a little easier while she was in another state.

Ultimately, fostering independence in your child is about trusting their abilities, trusting their resilience, and trusting that the foundation you have built together will support them as they take these next steps. Independence isn't a destination but a journey that you and your child will navigate together. As they grow into young adults, your relationship will evolve, and in that evolution lies the beauty of watching them become the person they're meant to be – confident, capable and uniquely themselves.

Learning to let go as your neurodivergent child becomes a young adult is one of the most challenging yet essential steps in your parenting journey – it's one I have particularly struggled with. It's natural to worry about how they will navigate a world that often feels indifferent, or even hostile, to their unique ways of being. However, letting go doesn't mean abandoning your support. Rather, it's about shifting your role from protector to ally, from manager to coach, from parent to friend and biggest cheerleader, and allowing them the space to explore their independence while knowing you will always be there if they stumble. It requires embracing the uncertainty of this new chapter and accepting that growth often comes from the struggle. The process is as much about your own growth as it is theirs, and you learning to take little steps back, watching on with a heart bursting with love and pride, as they begin to write the pages of their own story.

Navigating challenges

Supporting your neurodivergent child into adulthood requires a commitment to remain calm and patient, even when the journey is challenging. As they navigate this complex transition there will absolutely be moments of frustration, setback and uncertainty – both for them and for you. By staying composed and offering consistent support, you will create an environment in which they feel safe and supported to grow at their own pace. This approach not only helps them build confidence but also models the self-regulation skills they will need throughout their adult life.

Supporting your young adult through struggles starts with being present and empathetic. It's important to acknowledge that their challenges may look different from those of their siblings or peers, and the way they react to problems might be unique to their neurodivergence. Instead of rushing to offer solutions, start by listening – really listening – to what they are experiencing and how they are feeling. Validate their emotions, letting them know that it's okay – and a regular part of being human – to struggle. Remind them that asking for help is a strength and not a weakness. Whether you assist them to find professional support, brainstorm coping strategies together, or simply make yourself available as a comforting presence, your support is about empowering them to face their struggles with resilience and self-compassion.

Sometimes, of course, you absolutely *will* need to jump in and take over the whole situation immediately, and that, too, is okay. One of the first times Chloé caught the train to Melbourne alone, she ran into trouble with ticket inspectors. She had purchased a concession ticket, but when they asked to see her concession card, she said she didn't have one. (She, of course, had a *student* card, but that's not what they asked her for – remember, autistic people often have very literal minds.)

These two big angry men in uniform then instructed her to hop off the train at the next stop, so they could take her in to an interview room *alone* and issue a fine. Our girl was absolutely terrified and confused about what she had done wrong. She panicked, had a shutdown *and* a meltdown, becoming unable to even speak to the officers. Of course, these men – who had *zero* training in neurodivergence – mistook her reaction as guilt and became very threatening towards her. This was all because of about a $3 difference in fare, I might add. Thankfully, Chloé was able to call me, and I demanded she put these men on the phone immediately. I growled like a mama bear down the phone at them and followed it up with a lengthy complaint to their management.

Needless to say, this episode caused far more damage to Chloé than it should have, and two years passed before she had the courage to catch the train alone again. But during that time, we made some communication cards for her that were helpful in explaining what tickets she may need, the language that ticket inspectors might use, and her rights and responsibilities as a passenger. It doesn't necessarily mean the same thing won't happen again, but hopefully Chloé will be better prepared if it does.

From Chloé 🦋

I still find adulting scary, but a loving family and comforting support tools make all the difference. If you're looking for me, I will be in my room watching *The Simpsons* and chatting with Peter Pan.

Adulting building blocks

Supporting your neurosparkly child into adulthood without damaging their self-esteem involves a delicate balance of encouragement, respect and understanding. It's best to honour their journey, recognise their strengths and celebrate their achievements (no matter how small or seemingly insignificant). Avoid comparing their progress to that of their neurotypical peers – or even worse, their siblings – as this can undermine their confidence and make them feel inadequate. Instead focus on their unique path and the personal growth they are experiencing.

Getting a driver's licence

Learning to drive can be one of the most exciting and significant milestones for all young adults. It is pretty much expected that as soon as you are allowed, you will go and get your licence. Tick.

However, for many people it is not that easy. I also always say having a driver's licence is a huge privilege and an even bigger responsibility – it's not your automatic right. It is imperative that you and your child feel ready for them to start to drive. Just because they can doesn't mean they should. (Come to think of it, there are probably plenty of 50-year-olds who shouldn't have their licence, either!)

Driving can present unique challenges for neurodivergent individuals, as it often requires multitasking, managing sensory inputs and responding quickly to changing situations. For those with ADHD, maintaining focus and staying organised while navigating can be difficult. Autistic individuals may struggle with processing complex visual information or handling sensory overload from traffic noise and lights. Additionally, executive function difficulties can impact tasks such as planning routes or remembering to check blind spots. Understanding these challenges is vital for developing strategies that support safe and confident driving, such as using adaptive tools, creating structured routines or seeking specialised driving instruction.

When supporting your child through the process, the best thing is to start talking about driving before they even think about applying for a learner's licence. You can narrate the things you are doing whenever you're in the car together. For example, I found myself constantly saying out loud, 'Even as we approach a green light at an intersection, I always look at each crossroads to make sure no one is accidentally running a red light,' so it would stick in my kids' heads.

A good driving instructor who is patient, kind and understands the unique needs of neurodivergent learners can be invaluable. If your child has an occupational therapist, they can also be really helpful with strategies for learning to drive. Break down driving lessons into manageable steps and practise in quiet areas before moving on to challenging environments. Encourage your child to take their time to feel comfortable behind the wheel, and remind them it's okay to take things more slowly and ask for extra help if needed. Using visual aids such as an approved GPS can help make navigation less overwhelming. I struggle with directions (an ADHD trait, I believe), and even if I have gone somewhere ten times before, I am likely to forget or get lost, so I always plug the address into my GPS before I leave.

Some people are simply not ready to get behind a wheel in their teens, and this is okay, too. We accepted that Chloé was not ready to drive after her sixth accident in her first year of driving. In the last one, she got totalled by a tram and could have lost her life, when she mistook a green light for hers when it was only for the tram. That day, when she rang me hysterically saying she'd had another accident, we realised it was just too unsafe for her to continue – for her and my heart. So she took a few years off driving altogether. She has recently gone back to short trips, and her confidence and ability have increased enormously.

It is also just fine to make the decision to never get your licence. This is why we have Ubers and public transport! My incredible grandmother went her entire life – well into her eighties and with four children – and never got her driver's licence.

When I asked her why, she simply said, 'I have never had any desire to drive, so I just made sure I married a man who did and spent my entire life being chauffeured around.' My grandma was a *very* smart woman!

Getting and keeping a job

Navigating the job market can be an exciting, scary and challenging part of neurodivergent adulthood. Autistic people have much higher rates of unemployment or underemployment than neurotypical people, and those with ADHD also report challenges with maintaining employment. But finding and keeping a job can be successful with the right support, tools and attitude.

The first step is to find a job that aligns with your child's passions, strengths and interests – ultimately, it's like matching a superhero with their ideal superpower. Walk into any gaming store, and I can almost guarantee that every one of the staff is neurodivergent. When you engage with them, their knowledge and expertise are infectious. You can see they genuinely love their job, and why wouldn't they?

When it comes to getting the job they want, practice makes perfect. Mock interviews and resume tweaks can turn nerves into confidence. Encourage your young adult to embrace their own unique skills and quirks as assets rather than obstacles. Building and maintaining a career often means mastering the art of communication – whether that's clarifying job expectations or handling workplace rules with grace. A good occupational therapist or psychologist can help with some of these skills. This might also be a good time to work on appropriate hygiene standards, dress-code expectations and anything else you think your child may need support with.

Prior to starting the job, it is helpful to build up your young adult's schedule to closely match that of their workplace. So if they are used to going to bed at midnight and then gaming for a few hours before waking up at midday, but they will now need to be up at 6 am for their new job, support them to transition over a period of weeks, if possible, to get their body clock used to this new rhythm.

Practise how they will get to the job. If this is by car, you may want to drive the route with them, show them where to park and how to access their workplace. If they will be using public transport, a practice run can help prepare them.

If they are taking their own lunch, figure out what they will feel comfortable eating at work and support them to choose what they will take.

Work uniforms, like school uniforms, can be uncomfortable and not sensory friendly. If they are required to wear them, encourage them to try them on and wear them in as best they can before their first day.

It can be helpful to have some discussions around small talk, current affairs and local news to get them ready for the 'watercooler chats' that are inevitable in many workplaces.

Once they're on the job, encourage them to communicate their needs clearly and professionally. Remind them that every job has its ups and downs, and that it's okay to ask for support or accommodations to help smooth the ride. It is also important to explain that in this day and age, it is unusual to stay in the same career for your entire work life – so it's fine to experiment. These days, the average young person will have up to seven different careers in their lifetime, and it is important your child understands that it is okay to move around, and if they leave or get fired, it's not the end of the world. With a positive mindset, a bit of humour and a dash of professionalism, they can turn their job into a rewarding adventure rather than just a daily grind.

One of my clients, Emily, recently secured her first job. She found she was struggling with intense sensory sensitivities and difficulty concentrating in the open-plan office spaces, which were noisy and distracting. We spent some time discussing her needs, and I encouraged her to request accommodations such as a quieter workspace, permission to use noise-cancelling headphones during work hours and the flexibility to work from home one day a week, to break up the week. Additionally, I encouraged Emily to ask for clear written instructions and deadlines to help her manage her workload effectively. Her employer instantly agreed to all these modifications, which not only showed Emily how valued she was but also allowed her to perform at her best. These simple accommodations led to a more supportive and productive work environment, and would have taken very little effort from her employer but made an enormous difference to Emily.

Managing money

When it comes to managing money, all young adults can benefit from a few simple strategies to help them stay organised and reduce stress. It always amazes me that basic money management is never taught in schools – and yet we have to learn *algebra*? – and we are just expected to work it out when we are suddenly in charge of our own money. It can be particularly challenging for neurodivergent people to manage their money, especially us ADHDers who tend to be impulsive (case in point: I have had *four* parcels arrive this week alone, and some I barely remember ordering. I call this an 'ADHD shopping bender' – another one for the Urban Dictionary!). For autistic people, the complexity of budgeting, tracking expenses and handling unexpected costs can be overwhelming. Sensory overload from financial tasks, or environments such as noisy bank branches or confusing online platforms, can add to the stress.

One helpful approach is to find budgeting tools that match your young adult's learning style – whether that's a simple spreadsheet, an app with visual aids or a colour-coded notebook. Some great budgeting apps offer visual features and reminders, making it easier to keep track of expenses and income. Having separate accounts for different types of expenses, including rent, groceries and entertainment, can also help with financial planning by creating clear boundaries for spending. Setting up automatic payments for regular bills can reduce the stress of remembering due dates, and creating a weekly check-in routine to review their spending can help them stay on track.

Long before my husband and I knew we both had ADHD, when we first moved in together, we had absolutely no comprehension of managing money or budgeting. We would spend each week's pay as soon as it came in, forgetting that bills would become due long after our pay had been spent. We would put the bills on a credit card until that was maxed out, and then we would apply for another, and the cycle continued. After we had racked up tens of thousands of dollars in credit-card debt, we finally learned to set up automatic bill payments for every single one of our bills. It can be helpful to line up direct debits for the day after your young adult's pay goes in, too. Encourage them to start with small, manageable financial goals, such as sticking to a budget for a month or saving up for a special purpose, and celebrate their progress along the way.

One of the young men I work with, Kai, has ADHD. He had recently moved out of home and into his first share house with three of his friends. He got paid fortnightly, and he impulsively spent the majority of his first pay cheque on a new gaming headset and games, leaving him short on funds for his contribution to rent and bills. Needless to say, his flatmates were not happy when he could not cough up his share of the bills. When he realised his mistake, he immediately contacted the bank of mum and dad, asking them to cover the shortfall.

Kai's mum came to me quite anxious, as they did not have the money to bail him out. She was also concerned that if they did, he would automatically do the same next fortnight – as he had always had problems with impulsivity and overspending – and they would then be left picking up the pieces every time this happened.

We sat down together and worked out a budget and a plan, organising a direct debit to come out of each pay to cover the essentials, so he would not even have access to this money. We then discussed ways Kai may be able to repay his debt or find additional money to cover this fortnight. Kai identified that he might be able to pick up some extra shifts at work, or sell some of his unwanted and unused games and gaming consoles, to cover the money his parents would loan him to get him out of trouble. This experience, while stressful, taught Kai the importance of financial responsibility and thinking ahead, skills that would serve him well in managing his future finances. It also alleviated the burden on his parents. It's important to remind your young adult that asking for help is okay if they feel overwhelmed, as seeking guidance is a valuable part of learning to manage money effectively.

Tertiary education

In my experience, tertiary education often turns out to be much better than high school for neurodivergent children, and here is why: it's all about freedom, fit and special interests. Unlike the rigid structure of high school, which often involves uncomfortable scratchy uniforms, long days, lots of rules and compulsory subjects, tertiary education allows your child to choose courses that actually interest them, play to their strengths and wear what they want. They also have more control over their schedule, which can help with managing sensory overload or energy dips.

Universities and colleges tend to have far better support systems in place, from disability services to student-led neurodivergent and neuro-affirming communities, offering a sense of belonging your child might have missed out on in high school. It's a time when they can truly embrace their individuality, find their tribe and thrive in an environment that respects and nurtures their unique way of learning and being in the world.

The other incredible benefit of tertiary education is the flexibility it offers. Most providers these days allow students to choose to be on campus, off campus or a blend of the two. They can also choose to be full-time or part-time, and as I often remind the students I work with, it is better to get there slowly and surely than to burn out from attempting to go full-time. 'How do you eat an elephant? One bite at a time!' meaning that if they break the course down into teeny tiny blocks of study – even if it is one subject at a time – they will eventually get there.

Giving support to your neurodivergent child through their tertiary studies is a bit like being their cheerleader, coach and occasional snack provider all rolled into one – not that different to high school, really. To set them up for success, encourage them to put the following supports in place:

- taking advantage of any resources available from disability inclusion units, such as extended time for exams, tutoring or notetaking services
- breaking down monstrous assignments into small bite-sized pieces – like slicing up a giant pizza
- using task apps, electronic calendars – or just a huge whiteboard on their bedroom wall – to keep track of their schedule and due dates
- colour-coding subject folders, books and other materials to keep them organised.

Regularly check in with your child, and offer to help out with managing time or prioritising tasks. But be mindful not to take over, instead focusing on empowering them to problem-solve and advocate for themselves.

One of the young adults I work with, Mia, struggled with time management during her first year of university. She had gone straight after finishing high school and had chosen not to advise the university that she is autistic and dyslexic. After missing several assignment deadlines, Mia was feeling so overwhelmed that she was considering dropping out, despite desperately wanting to do this course and absolutely being capable of doing so with the right support.

Her mum was so concerned that she wanted to contact the university on Mia's behalf to advise the course director of Mia's diagnoses. I explained this was not her role, no matter how much the mama bear in her wanted to intervene. Instead, we sat down with Mia and encouraged her to take a step back and assess her priorities. We reminded her how much she had wanted to get into this course. We discussed how beneficial the disability inclusion unit at university was, and that by reaching out to them,

Mia would be able to get the additional support and understanding she needed to successfully complete the course. We discussed that the university offering her some extra support was no different from them providing a wheelchair ramp for a wheelchair user, and that she had nothing to be ashamed of.

I then unpacked why Mia was hesitant to advise the university of her support needs. She admitted that even though her high-school classmates had been aware of her diagnoses, she wanted to start fresh with university. This, of course, was her right. When I explained that the university had a legal obligation to keep this confidential from anyone other than her teachers, she agreed to contact them.

We then spent some time looking on the university website to work out how Mia would go about contacting them online. We also identified appropriate apps and planners that could be beneficial to her and offered guidance on how she could use those to her advantage.

Mia contacted the disability unit herself, and I provided her with a letter explaining her diagnoses and the support she required. The disability unit staff then scheduled an online meeting with Mia to discuss her accommodations, which included having extra time to complete tasks and a learning adviser to look over her work for spelling mistakes and grammatical errors before she submitted it. As expected, they were incredibly supportive of Mia, and she felt a lot more motivated to continue. This experience empowered Mia to take control of her responsibilities and trust her own capacity to overcome challenges and also advocate for herself, all without mama bear having to get directly involved.

I often remind my students that 'Even Ps get degrees' (where the P stands for 'pass'). Many of the neurodivergent people

I have worked with are really high achievers and perfectionists, so they can be super hard on themselves and will aim for high distinctions or 100 per cent on everything. Unlike in high school, where actual marks can be important, once you are in university, whether you get 50 per cent or 100 per cent, you get the same piece of paper at the end. So it may be better for them to try to lower their standards to reduce those stress levels.

Socialising

Socialising can be both exciting and challenging (and nerve-racking) for young neurodivergent adults, but with some practical tips, lots of love and a supportive environment, they can build meaningful connections.

Safe social spaces

Encourage them to start by exploring social situations that align with their interests, such as joining a club, a gaming group or an online community where they can meet others who share their passions. It can also help to practise social scenarios in advance, role-playing different conversations to boost their confidence and prepare them for various situations. Remind them that it's okay to take breaks during social activities when they feel overwhelmed, and that setting boundaries is important for their wellbeing. Highlight the value of quality over quantity in friendships (boy, don't we realise this one as we get older?), emphasising that meaningful connections are about finding people who appreciate and accept them for who they are.

One of the ways we supported Chloé's socialising in a safe place – and have gone on to do this with all of our kids – was for our home to become known as the party house. Now, party house and neurodivergent kids don't necessarily sound like the best match, but for our kids who do want to be social and attend parties occasionally, it can be so much easier and more supportive to do that in your own environment. It also gives our kids the opportunity to learn how to party like an adult in the safety of our own home.

For several years once Chloé turned eighteen, we held a New Year's Eve party at our house for her friends – most of whom were the young adults she had become friends with in the social group she had been attending. They were all neurodivergent and all struggled socially. The thought of them all going out to night-clubs in town, especially on New Year's Eve, sent shivers down my spine. So we decided to make the best New Year's Eve parties that anyone had ever seen, and we became quite famous for them. Thinking of all of these glorious young adults, covered in glow sticks and drinking their favourite drinks while dancing the

SARAH'S THREE TOP TIPS FOR NEURODIVERGENT YOUNG ADULT SOCIALISING

1. Start small: begin with low-pressure social situations, such as a small gathering or a one-on-one meet-up, to build confidence gradually.

2. Find shared interests: encourage them to join clubs, groups or online communities centred around their hobbies. It is so much easier to connect when you share common interests. Dungeons & Dragons, anyone?

3. Practice makes perfect: role-play different social scenarios at home to make them feel prepared. Practise greetings, small talk and how to politely end a conversation (or leave a party they don't want to be at).

night away, still brings a smile to my face. Remember, this is a learning experience and there will be mistakes made at these parties – our job is to sit quietly, away from the party but close enough to be on call if needed. If you are lucky – as we were – you might even get invited to join them.

Romantic relationships

Marriage – or a long-term relationship – is arguably the most significant life milestone, which comes with its own set of challenges for everyone. But for neurosparkly people these challenges can be unique and complex, given how confusing they can find social interactions to be.

Supporting your young adult child to developing mature, long-lasting relationships involves fostering self-awareness, communication skills and emotional resilience. Encourage them to understand their own needs and boundaries while also respecting those of others. Help them practise clear and honest communication, and offer guidance on navigating social dynamics and conflict resolution. Providing opportunities for social interaction in comfortable settings can build their confidence. Emphasise the importance of mutual respect and understanding in relationships, and support them in finding communities or support groups where they can build meaningful connections, while honouring their uniquely neurodivergent perspective. It is likely that, even as an adult, your child will need additional guidance and support to navigate each step of the relationship.

One of my clients, a young woman named Susan, came to me distressed by relationship difficulties. She had recently moved into the home of her partner, whom she adored, and they were suddenly having a lot of fights, which had never happened prior to them living together. He was annoyed that when he came home from work, she did not appear excited to see him, and she didn't speak to him or hug him. He read this as her being angry with him or uninterested in how his day had been. But, in fact, having worked in a noisy childcare centre all day, Susan was absolutely exhausted and in sensory overload, needing a couple of hours to reset before she could even talk to – let alone touch – another person. Until we unpacked this, even Susan had not realised why she was responding in this way.

Helping Susan understand how her brain works allowed her to share these insights with her partner so they could work on their relationship. He decided to go straight from work to the gym each afternoon, giving her time alone at home to decompress and reset. This extra time gave her the ability to genuinely give him the response he craved when he got home to see her. Honest, open communication is the key to resolving most relationship issues.

Surviving a wedding

Of course, one of the most joyous parts of marriage is the wedding. Since Chloé's wedding, I have had so many people reach out to me, asking me how she coped and what we did to make things easier. Let's be honest: a wedding day can be hard and stressful for even the most neurotypical of people!

My little Tinkerbell, who had never wanted to grow up, get married or move out of home, was getting married. For anyone who has looked at pictures and footage, you'll have seen that the wedding was utterly spectacular and perfect, so beyond our wildest dreams. What you won't have seen are the meltdowns leading up to the wedding, the meltdowns on the day of the wedding, the tears dotted in between the incredibly happy moments of the day, and the comedown afterward, which lasted for weeks.

A few days before the wedding, Chloé tried her dress on. It was stunningly beautiful, like something out of a Disney princess movie, and it was also heavy and scratchy and uncomfortable and tight and hard. There were tears from her, then tears from me, and then undoubtedly tears from the designers, who had worked tirelessly to create this piece of art. The dress was absolutely on point for fashion, but not sensory friendly for a girl who has huge sensory needs. Thankfully we had the most *amazing* and patient and wonderful designers, who worked around the clock for the next 48 hours to transform the dress into not only the most superb gown, but also the soft, comfortable, sensory-friendly dress of Chloé's dreams. They lined it with the softest of satins, took out the boning, removed the weight and had it softly tied with the prettiest of ribbons, which were gentle on her delicate skin. She also wore her favourite, most comfortable western boots under the dress.

We ensured all the dishes served at the wedding were Chloé's favourites, with her special snacks and drinks scattered in places she could access easily. Every now and then one of her safe people would whisk her away to check in on her, give her a breather if she needed it and remind her that tomorrow wasn't going to be any different than yesterday. While she never had a single doubt that she was marrying the man of her dreams, and never had a moment of questioning if she was doing the right thing, she *also* didn't want anything to change. I think the biggest relief for all of us was when she woke up the day after her wedding and said, 'Nothing feels any different than it did before I got married.' Phew!

Moving out of home

You get married and then you move out of home. That's the way it goes for most people, if they don't already have their own home. And the expectation is that once you buy a house, you move straight into it. But, with our neurodivergent kids, it's vital to let go of societal expectations. You can simply take things as they come without judgement. Your child is in charge of their own life, so they get to make the rules. Who says you have to buy a house and move straight in? For Chloé, it took a lot more time to prepare for and transition into this new phase of life.

Supporting your neurodivergent child as they prepare to move out of home involves a thoughtful approach that blends practical preparation with emotional readiness. This process should be paced according to their own comfort level, ensuring they feel empowered rather than overwhelmed. Alongside the practicalities of budgeting and developing routines, it's important to address the emotional aspect of transitioning into living independently, including talking about their hopes, fears and expectations. Reassure them that moving out of home doesn't mean losing your support; rather, it's a new chapter in which your relationship evolves and you continue to be there for guidance and encouragement. By equipping them with the skills they need and fostering a positive outlook on this significant and exciting life change, you help them approach this milestone with confidence and a sense of excitement for the independence ahead.

The first step for Chloé was buying a home just down the road from our family home – literally two kilometres away. It's close enough that she can come over every single day if she wants. Close enough that we are always there if she needs us, *when* she needs us. Close enough that I can run her favourite comfort food, my lentil dhal, down to her on a bad day or when every other food just tastes wrong. Close enough that if the world is just too much for her, we are there. Close enough that if she feels the need to spend more time at the family home and less time at her home, she can.

The second step was a very slow transition. Most people pack up all their stuff and move in a day. For Chloé, it has taken more than twelve months so far . . . and counting. The thought of packing up 26 years of childhood toys and memories into boxes, leaving her room and setting up a new house all at once was just too much to bear. So it's been a gradual, careful move. A box here and a box there, bit by bit and hardly noticeable. Then sleepovers at the new house. Shower and PJs on at the family home, then down to her house for a sleepover, then back to the family home first thing the next day for breakfast and to spend the day. Eventually, it will be longer days at the new house and less time here, but there is absolutely no hurry. Transitions can be really hard for our kids, so allow them to take the time they need.

Once they're in their own place, parenting from afar requires a careful balance of giving your neurosparkly children space to grow while remaining a reliable source of support. Even if you're not physically present, your connection can remain strong through regular meaningful communication that reassures them they are not alone and you are still very much a part of their journey. Whether it's regular phone calls, video chats or texts (or even sending some groceries, Uber Eats or a cleaner around), staying in touch as much as you can helps maintain the bond you have built over the years. It is important to respect their autonomy and trust in their ability to manage their life, offering them advice and guidance when asked, rather than stepping in uninvited. When challenges arise, be there to listen and help them problem-solve but also allow them the dignity of finding their own solutions. By showing confidence and support in their independence, while offering a consistent compassionate presence, you'll help them navigate adulthood with the knowledge that they have a solid support system.

Q & A

Q: MY SON HAS ADHD. SHOULD HE DISCLOSE THIS IN A JOB INTERVIEW?

A: While we should always be neuro-affirming and proud of who we are, with nothing to hide, unfortunately, the whole world does not yet see us like this. So while I would love to say, 'Hell yes, rock up to your job interview with *PROUDLY AND LOUDLY ADHD* emblazoned across your t-shirt for all to see,' I will actually say I think it's better to secure the job first. Then, if you feel it is necessary to disclose, and accommodations are needed, you can contact your manager or HR to discuss.

If you feel you need accommodations for the job interview, it's important to advocate for yourself early in the process. Reach out to the employer ahead of time, ideally when the interview is scheduled, and explain the accommodations that would help you perform at your best. These might include having extra time for answering questions, receiving the interview format in advance or conducting the interview in a quiet, sensory-friendly environment. Most employers are legally required to provide reasonable accommodations, and being upfront about your needs helps ensure the process is more comfortable, setting the stage for a successful interview. Additionally, this will show you if your potential employer is willing and able to make the adjustments you may require if you are successful in securing the job.

Q: MY DAUGHTER IS AUTISTIC AND IS PREPARING TO MOVE OUT OF HOME. WHAT ARE SOME PRACTICAL TIPS TO HELP HER MANAGE DAILY TASKS AND RESPONSIBILITIES EFFECTIVELY?

A: Supporting your daughter through the transition to move out is a huge step for both of you. Some practical tips include:

- Create structured routines with clear visual schedules.
- Use checklists and visual reminders to help her stay organised and remember important tasks, such as meal planning, cleaning, and managing money and appointments.
- Break down tasks into smaller manageable steps to make them less overwhelming. For example, instead of trying to clean the entire house, she can break it down into small tasks such as: pick up all your dirty laundry, put a load of washing on, collect all the dirty dishes, put a dishwasher load on, and so on.
- Download helpful organising tools and apps.
- Establish a designated space for important items such as keys, bills and documents to help reduce stress and confusion. Labelling boxes and having a place for everything can be really helpful in reducing stress and maintaining the home, which we know can be a struggle for neurodivergent people . . . especially if Mum's not on hand to help out.

Q: MY NEURODIVERGENT SON STRUGGLES WITH FRIENDSHIPS AND FINDS SOCIAL SITUATIONS EXTREMELY OVERWHELMING, BUT IS ALSO LONELY AND ISOLATED SINCE FINISHING SCHOOL. I WANT TO HELP HIM BUILD HIS SOCIAL SKILLS AND ENSURE HE IS NOT LIVING AS A TOTAL HERMIT. WHAT ARE SOME PRACTICAL TIPS I CAN USE TO SUPPORT HIM?

A: Start by encouraging him to identify and engage in activities that he already enjoys, especially those that involve group settings such as a club or hobby group. This way he can meet others who share his special interests, which will make socialising easier and more natural. Many of the young men I work with love gaming, so they have found either online or face-to-face gaming groups and connected with fellow gamers this way. There are so many wonderful options on social media now – a quick search will uncover just about any special-interest group.

If you can't find a suitable group for your young adult, start one! We found the best way for our kids to socialise was opening up our house to their friends, and it was so much fun. Knowing they were safe and comfortable in their own home was worth any amount of time and effort we ever had to put in to any party or gathering we held.

You can also practise social scenarios together at home, which helps build confidence before he's out in real life situations. Role-playing, for example, can be particularly helpful – you can have him practise introducing himself or asking someone about their day.

Another key point is to help him set boundaries, including letting him know it's okay to take breaks during social activities or to leave early if he is feeling overwhelmed. We taught all of our kids if they wanted to leave anywhere, at any time, for any reason, they could just text us and say 'you want me to come home', and we would then text or call immediately, apologising, saying we needed them to come home for whatever reason. It was their get-out-of-jail-free card that blamed us, not them, for leaving.

Chapter 9

Adult diagnosis

For many parents, going through the process of their child receiving a diagnosis of autism, ADHD or another type of neurodivergence leads them to question whether they, too, may be neurodivergent. For some, pursuing a diagnosis for themselves can bring a sense of relief, an explanation as to why they have always felt different. For others, it means they can get practical or financial support, or be better understood in the workplace or university, or within their family and friendship group. Some adults choose to self-identify as neurodivergent without an official diagnosis, which – just like with kids – is widely accepted by the neurosparkly community. Coming to understand your own neurodivergence may even have the added perk of giving you more insight into how your child's brain works.

If you, your partner or your grown-up children are considering seeking an adult diagnosis, welcome to the club. As someone who's had three members of my family (including myself) be first diagnosed as adults, let me walk you through it.

From Chloé and Ronnie 🦋

I'm going to leave this one to my dad, Ronnie, who was diagnosed at 49. While his diagnosis was no surprise to me, I think he is best to tell that story:

Getting diagnosed at 49 with autism, ADHD and dyslexia was a strange experience. Knowing how awesome Chloé is meant that I didn't see autism as a negative diagnosis. Instead, I just thought, I'm part of the club. However, over the next few months I began to mourn for myself as a young boy who was so misunderstood. I wish I could find a time machine, go back 40 years and have one or two people in my life read this chapter. It excites me that this book is out now. The more people who understand neurosparkly minds, the earlier people will be diagnosed and feel supported.

Coming late to diagnosis

While receiving a diagnosis as an adult can be a relief, it can also bring about many mixed feelings, including shame, embarrassment, confusion, joy, sadness, regret . . . all of which are fine, perfectly normal and to be expected.

For me, receiving a diagnosis of ADHD at the age of 48 was a roller-coaster of emotions. It was while sitting in on Chloé's ADHD assessment that I realised I, too, ticked every single box for ADHD. This was a light-bulb moment: she and I were similar in so many ways because our brains were made up of the same amazing, sparkly glitter. When I sat through her final appointment, where her diagnosis was confirmed, I actually asked the assessing psychologist (jokingly, but not really) if he could also provide me with a diagnosis. Sadly – and unsurprisingly – he said no. It was worth a shot!

A few more years down the track, I finally decided to invest the time and money to officially pursue my own diagnosis, even though I was sure of the answer. I had struggled with feeling different for years, always wondering why some things seemed so much harder for me than for others. Getting an official diagnosis was like unlocking a door to self-understanding. It gave me the language to describe my experiences and helped me feel validated, not broken. Knowing I am neurodivergent allowed me to make sense of the ways I process the world. It's not about labels; it's about *self-awareness, understanding, acceptance and empowerment*, giving me the tools to thrive in a society that wasn't built with my brain in mind.

We know that autism and ADHD tend to run in families, so if your child has been diagnosed, there's a good chance at least one of the parents will be, too. Whenever I talk to parents about this, I see them looking at each other trying to work out who passed it on. It used to be almost a blame game, but these days it's more like a claim to fame! Well, as it turns out, in our family it was both parents (more on this below) – so I guess the odds of Chloé being neurodivergent were pretty high.

Not long after receiving her ADHD diagnosis, plus having already been diagnosed with dyslexia in high school, my beautiful 22-year-old daughter Gemma also received a diagnosis of autism. To say I felt badly is an understatement. To miss that diagnosis for that long when I was an autism professional who educated people on autism, and had already been through the process with my first-born, made me feel like a pretty crappy mum.

So if you are feeling bad about a late diagnosis, please don't. There is such a huge variation in how neurodivergence presents – my two eldest daughters couldn't be more different, and yet they are both autistic with ADHD. Like many autistic women, Gemma had learned to hide the signs of autism to fit in. She was an exceptional copycat and extremely high masker who appeared to cope very well with social situations. It was overwhelming anxiety that eventually led to her autism diagnosis. She was the typical little duck in the pond – appearing calm and gliding along on the surface but paddling furiously underwater just to stay afloat. We all need to acknowledge our efforts beneath the surface to promote a culture of transparency – one in which asking for help, revealing our hidden struggles and seeking support are not seen as signs of weakness or failure but rather courageous steps towards discovering who we really are and what we need.

When I finally received my own official diagnosis, I swung between feeling sad it had taken me 48 years to find out and regret for all those years when I could have understood my brain better. I particularly reflected on how my childhood could have been so much more positive had I, and others around me, understood me better. But ultimately I was happy, excited, proud and so relieved that I had received the diagnosis that not only gave me life membership to a pretty cool club, but also gave me – and those around me – the permission and the tools to better understand myself, and *be* myself.

Getting an official diagnosis as an adult can feel overwhelming, but it's a powerful step towards understanding yourself better. Start by reaching out to a professional such as a psychologist or a psychiatrist who specialises in neurodivergence. You can ask your primary-care provider for a referral or do some research to find experts who focus on adults. There are many, many clinics set up solely for the purposes of autism and ADHD assessments. They can vary a lot in wait times and price, so it's well worth doing some research. The process usually involves interviews, questionnaires and assessments of your personal and medical history. Be prepared for it to take time (and money), but remember, this is about gaining insight and access to the right support. The diagnosis can open doors to accommodations and resources, and, most importantly, a deeper sense of self-awareness. I want to add that – again, in Australia, at least – if you are wanting to trial medications for ADHD, you will need a diagnosis from a psychiatrist, rather than a psychologist's assessment, to access those medications.

If you do get diagnosed as an adult, some people in your life may question its validity. Many adults who are in the public eye and late diagnosed are slammed on social media for 'coming out' (look at what Em Rusciano went through) and asked why they suddenly 'appear' neurodivergent, or to be more obviously struggling, when they never have before. People will actually say things such as, 'You never used to be autistic!' As if you suddenly woke up one day and decided to spend thousands of dollars seeking an assessment just for fun.

The real answer is simple. When you are younger, you may have had more support and more capacity to handle life, as well as less pressure and more time to decompress. The older you get, the more there is going on, especially if you are a parent – work stress, kids, financial pressures, no downtime, expectations to meet neurotypical adult standards . . . the list goes on.

So people may ask if you are 'faking it' now, but the truth is you were probably 'faking it' before. And faking it, or masking, is only going to end in burnout, mental health issues and depression. Also . . . who the hell gave them permission to question *your* diagnosis? No one needs those people in their life. Don't ever let anyone question you or your diagnosis: no one has this right.

Some other people may ask, 'Why bother getting a diagnosis now?' Getting my diagnosis as an adult changed everything for me. It was like finally seeing the full picture after years of missing pieces. I stopped blaming myself for things I struggled with and started understanding why my brain works the way it does. It allowed me to embrace my strengths (and sparkles!) and find strategies to manage my challenges. More than anything, though, it gave me a sense of peace and validation – finally knowing there wasn't anything 'wrong' with me, just that I process the world differently. It opened up new possibilities and new connections with others who share similar experiences, including my own husband and children, and it set me on a new career path. It truly changed the way I live my life – for me, it was nothing but positive.

While writing this book I received a text from an adult friend telling me she had just been diagnosed autistic, and how it was a lot to take in and process. After first congratulating her on her awesomeness, I reminded her that she hasn't *just* been diagnosed, but, rather, she has just *discovered* why her brain works the way it does, and now she can better understand it. How cool is that? And don't we all deserve to fully understand and accept ourselves just as we are?

Revisiting childhood trauma

This section mentions sexual assault, so please go gently (or avoid if you need to).

The adult diagnosis process will require you to delve into your childhood, since neurodivergence is a lifelong presentation. This may bring up uncomfortable memories or trauma. While I am now confidently and unashamedly a sparkly, glittery MGT – or Mama Glitter Tits, as some in Chloé's community have christened me – who wears giant loud earrings, sadly, I wasn't always this way.

My childhood was difficult in many ways. Looking back, I can see all the signs of ADHD that were missed at the time. I was always the kid who couldn't sit still, constantly daydreaming when I was supposed to be paying attention. My mind would race, jumping from one thought to the next, and I often (always) struggled to follow through on tasks, even when I wanted to. I'd lose things constantly – homework, toys, you name it – and always forgot what I was supposed to be doing. People called me scatterbrained or a daydreamer, but really I was just overwhelmed. Now I realise these moments were part of my neurodivergent wiring, not a failure to try hard enough, as I was sometimes made to feel.

My teenage years were especially horrendous. I went to an elite all-girls private school and I didn't fit in with *any* of the girls. I wandered between groups, trying desperately to be accepted, but I never was. I was constantly changing like a chameleon yet never able to find the right pattern. A desperate need to fit in led me to some questionable behaviour, such as dyeing my hair 'black cherry' and graffitiing my books with 'The Cure' to mimic the new goth girl at school.

When I was just fourteen, a boy from our brother school took an interest in me. Given that none of the girls would even sit with me at lunchtime, let alone hang out on the weekends, I gravitated to this boy like a moth to a flame. I now realise he was probably a predator who saw my naivety and vulnerability as easy to exploit. I had an insatiable appetite to be loved and accepted, no matter what it cost.

That cost would turn out to be unacceptably high. During my teen years, I would suffer multiple sexual assaults and an ongoing relationship of abuse. My desperate need to please and my lack of friends put a glowing neon light on my forehead that said, 'I have no self-esteem, and I have no one to protect me.' I was an obvious target. Research tells us that those with autism and ADHD are much more likely to be sexually assaulted. One study showed that autistic girls have almost three times the risk of being coerced into sex, while girls with ADHD have double the risk. Neurodivergent boys are also at more risk of sexual assault than neurotypical boys.

Neurodivergent girls may have trouble understanding social norms or recognising dangerous situations. Lifelong masking also teaches us to focus entirely on what is the expected response – the people-pleasing response – instead of listening to our own senses, needs and desires. It is so much easier to manipulate someone with low self-esteem who is constantly trying to act the way they 'should', especially when girls are taught we must be good and obedient.

Looking back on my teen years through the lens of neurodivergence was painful, but it also allowed me to extend more kindness and compassion to little Sarah. If you are battling similar trauma, I hope that sharing this will help you to feel less alone, and know that you will receive endless love and support in the neurodivergent community. The hope is that if we can address our own childhood traumas, we will be able to be more grounded and present for our children.

I know how confronting it can be to face the reality that our neurodivergent kids are at higher risk of sexual assault. As a parent, the best thing you can do is ensure that your child, whether neurodivergent or not, has as much education as possible, starting as early as possible, to protect them from abuse. Especially with neurodivergent kids, it's important to keep the information simple and direct about what behaviour is unacceptable. It is never too early – or late – to start these conversations, and it's helpful to revisit them regularly to keep the lines of communication open with your child so that they feel comfortable telling you about any incidents that arise. Every single child has the right to grow up free from abuse, and it is up to every adult to create a safe environment.

If you or someone you know is struggling with sexual abuse, please seek support (see page 290 for helpful resources).

Understanding your neurosparkly partner

When I booked myself in for my ADHD assessment, both my husband, Ronnie, and my second-eldest daughter, Gemma, asked if I could also book appointments for them. They already shared a diagnosis of dyslexia, but they suspected they also shared undiagnosed ADHD. The three of us were assessed by three different psychologists at the same clinic. That was an expensive day! We then had appointments on the same morning to receive our official results. It was no great surprise when the three of us texted each other to confirm our ADHD diagnoses.

What did come as a pretty big shock to me, however, was that Ronnie also walked out with a diagnosis of autism. He didn't text that part to me – he called me after the appointment to tell me. Funnily enough, he was not shocked at all to hear he was autistic, because over the years, whenever he had heard Chloé share her story or her struggles, he had realised his experiences were similar.

The thing about adult diagnosis is that if you have reached adulthood without understanding or addressing the challenges that your neurodivergence brings, it's likely that you will have developed particular coping mechanisms in your relationships that will need to be re-examined. This process can be particularly intense with long-term partners, who may have been unconsciously holding you to neurotypical standards and wondering why you're always falling short.

Receiving an adult diagnosis may make you realise that many of the coping mechanisms you've developed over the years aren't actually helping you. They are just ways you have learned to survive without fully understanding yourself. You may avoid conflict by shutting down, or masking your true feelings to fit in, thinking that's what you need to do to keep the peace. After a diagnosis, you can begin to unlearn those habits and replace them with healthier ways to communicate and connect. You learn that you don't have to hide who you are to be loved or understood. It's a process of relearning how to show up authentically in all relationships.

For me it was another *huge* light-bulb moment. Almost 30 years of living with Ronnie, this man I adored, whom I (thought I) knew better than anyone, flashed before my eyes. I now had a deeper understanding and appreciation of him and so many things we had gone through. I also felt sadness that

I had not realised it earlier so I could better understand him, and us. Throughout our entire relationship there had been so many little things he did that confused or frustrated me, and suddenly it all made perfect sense.

For example, if I texted Ronnie something like, 'Can you please grab some bread on the way home from work?' he would never reply. *Never*. I would then assume he hadn't read the message, and go out to get bread. He would come home with bread and ask why I had got some as well as asking him to get it. I would say, 'I assumed you didn't read my text as you didn't reply to me.' He would then say, 'I didn't realise you wanted a reply, I just thought you wanted bread. You never asked for a reply.' He was confused and I was confused. His diagnosis helped me realise that he needed more explicit directions, for example: 'Can you please grab some bread on the way home from work, and just let me know you got this message so I know I don't have to get bread.' Now I get a little thumbs up in response. Simple! Communication is everything.

Another thing Ronnie has always done is be early for everything. If a party starts at 6 pm and it takes fifteen minutes to drive there, we must be in the car *at least* twenty minutes prior to allow for fluctuating traffic conditions, because we must arrive before the stated time on the invite. I literally had to google 'party etiquette' to explain to him that it is socially *acceptable* to be fifteen minutes late to a party but socially *unacceptable* to be early. This has been a difficult one to navigate when you have my messy ADHD brain, which is always running late, competing with his autistic brain, which must be early. (Although *his* ADHD brain leaves his dirty washing on the floor!)

Even though Ronnie holds a job for which he frequently fronts the media, talks to rooms full of hundreds of people and runs large training seminars and conferences, he is incredibly uncomfortable making small talk or going places where he doesn't know people. It used to frustrate me that he never wanted to attend anything for me or my work, or for any of my friends he didn't know, but he was always fine with anything that related to him. I used to think he was being selfish but since his diagnosis, I now realise this stems from his intense social anxiety. He needs to feel secure and in control and know that he has something to talk about with other people (like a special interest, for example). Knowing this has made *such* a difference in our relationship.

I was so proud of my husband for sharing his diagnosis with his colleagues and staff, and even letting them know what support he needs from them. Even prouder to know the only reason he felt brave enough to do this is because he had spent so many years learning from his own daughter. *Wow.*

Let's return to those people who may question the point of a late diagnosis. I hope it has helped for me to explain what a difference a diagnosis has made for Ronnie and me, after 30 years together, to be able to adjust our communication style so that it works for both of us. If you truly love or care for someone, you should want to know everything about them, and this includes how we can ensure their needs are being met, as well as our own. If we don't truly understand the other person and how their brain works, it can be like we are each speaking a language that the other doesn't understand. Impossible!

Shifting these relationship patterns isn't an overnight process, of course. Navigating relationships after receiving an adult diagnosis of neurodivergence – whether your own or your partner's – can feel like daunting unchartered territory, but it can also be an opportunity for growth and deeper connection. By taking some practical steps, it can actually strengthen your bond.

Start by learning together. Read up on the diagnosis and explore how it may affect daily life, communication and emotional needs. This shared understanding helps create a foundation of empathy. Next, establish new routines or adjustments where needed. For example, if sensory sensitivities are an issue, you might adjust your living space to be more comfortable.

It's also crucial to check in regularly, so set aside time to discuss how things are going, and if any new strategies are helping or need tweaking. Remember, there is likely to be a grieving process for both people – receiving a diagnosis as an adult can be challenging to hear. Not because it's a bad thing, but it can be hard to know you have gotten to a certain age without knowing who you are and what support you really needed. Be open to seeking outside support, such as couples therapy with a neuro-affirming therapist, to help navigate the challenges together. Embrace the fact that this diagnosis can offer clarity and tools to make your relationship more adaptable and resilient.

Some things that bug you about your partner may stem from unmet needs, in which case a diagnosis can offer better understanding and support. These might include:

- Forgetting plans or important dates: this may come from difficulties with executive functioning or memory. A diagnosis can help explain the need for reminders or external organisation systems and stop you from attributing their behaviour to carelessness.

- Difficulty expressing emotions: understanding that your partner may struggle with emotional regulation, or have a different way of processing feelings, can highlight the need for clearer, more direct communication strategies.
- Needing alone time or retreating from social situations: this can stem from sensory overload or social exhaustion. A diagnosis helps frame this as a necessary recharge rather than a lack of interest in spending time together.
- Being hyperfocused on a task or hobby: this intense focus might be linked to how your partner's brain processes stimulation. Recognising this through a diagnosis shows they are not ignoring you, or choosing their hobby over you, but it's instead about how they manage their focus and energy.
- Rigid routine or resistance to change: this could come from a need for predictability to reduce anxiety. A diagnosis helps explain this as a coping mechanism, which can encourage you to take a more supportive approach when changes are unavoidable.

Understanding neurodivergence in a relationship can be transformative, offering new insights into behaviours that may have caused frustration in the past. A diagnosis provides clarity, revealing that many of these challenges stem from unmet needs rather than a lack of care or effort. With this knowledge, you can approach your partner with more empathy and adjust your expectations to fit their unique needs and strengths. Ultimately, this deeper understanding can foster healthier communication, greater patience and a stronger, more supportive relationship. It's not about fixing your partner; it's about learning to navigate life together with mutual respect and compassion.

Your time to shine

Interestingly, around the time I received my diagnosis, I started unashamedly covering myself in glitter when I went out – and Mama Glitter Tits was born. I also embraced wearing the earrings I had always loved and admired on other women but lacked the confidence to wear. Big, bold earrings with incredibly bright colours and sparkles that demand attention. The kind of earrings that, when I wear them now, other women stop me admiringly and say, 'Oh my gosh, I love your earrings! I always wanted to be the kind of woman to wear those earrings, but I just can't get away with it. But you absolutely can!' The kind of earrings that say, 'I am confident. I am comfortable in my own skin. I am not going to hide away or dull my sparkle.'

It was such a revelation that I had spent 48 years trying to make myself smaller, quieter, more demure. Suddenly I had permission to be myself. I was no longer going to deny myself the simple sparkly pleasures in life – it was my time to shine. Just as I had always encouraged my own kids to proudly and authentically be themselves, so, too, was I giving myself that permission.

And now I give *you* the same permission – glitter up, pop in those huge 'look at me' earrings, swipe on the bright red lipstick, wear the dopamine-rush candy-coloured clothes, or whatever else it is that you love but don't do for fear of being 'too much' . . . now it's *your* time to shine, baby!

Rediscovering your authentic self after your diagnosis is like peeling back layers you didn't even know were there. For years, you have likely been masking and adapting to fit into a world around you, trying to be what you think you should be. But once you receive a diagnosis, you can give yourself permission to explore who you really are beneath all of that.

Start by paying attention to what genuinely makes you happy, the environments where you thrive, your passions and strengths, and how you can honour your needs without guilt or shame. It's a journey of self-compassion, where you can learn to embrace the parts of yourself you once tried to hide. There is nothing more empowering than finally living authentically. It's about unlearning old patterns, embracing your neurodivergent traits and living in a way that feels the most true to who you are.

It has taken me a very long time, but since my diagnosis I can now recognise and celebrate my ADHD strengths, which I know are also admired by others. While I still struggle to make and keep friends, I have a very small but close-knit circle, and that's all I need.

My many awesome ADHD superpowers that benefit me daily include:

- Abundant energy: I have five kids, a busy, stressful full-time job, I study, I write, I volunteer *and* keep a clean house (I can't stand mess; it makes my head messy). Not to say I don't get exhausted sometimes – I do – but for the most part, I have enough energy to juggle all the balls and channel this towards success and a life I love. I get bored so quickly, so my brain needs constant stimulus and excitement. After all, a sparkly rainbow brain needs a sparkly rainbow life!
- Spontaneity: I love to keep things exciting and hate the mundane. I turn impulsivity into spontaneity, which makes me a pretty fun person to be around. It is not unusual for

me to suddenly buy a new car, a new dog, a new house, book a trip, sign up to a university degree . . . things that others think about for years I do on a whim . . . did someone say dopamine rush?

- Excitement and enthusiasm: I have such a zest for life. I get so excited about things that I get intense bursts of speed, enthusiasm and determination, all of which contribute to high energy levels to get all the things done. Admittedly, they're often done at the last minute, but still . . . all the things *do* get done.

- Creativity: my imaginative, busy and creative mind is always dreaming up new ideas and new ways to do things. I am original, artistic and creative.

- Ability to hyperfocus: I can become so intently focused on a task, I don't even notice what is going on around me. I have the ability to work on something until its completion without breaking concentration, even if it means going all night, not eating or having a toilet break . . . wait that's probably not *totally* a positive, is it?

I have so many awesome qualities and quirks that are highly valued and admired. Not a day goes by when people don't stop and ask me how I can do all I can do, nearly always with a smile on my face and a positive attitude. I am known as Super Mum (or MGT), and I am always asked my secrets. I used to shrug my shoulders and say humbly, 'Oh I don't know, it's just me,' but now I answer: 'ADHD is my superpower!' And it's the truth.

It's not all positive, of course. There are a few things I struggle with, such as time management (hi, and apologies to my editor!), concentration, staying on topic, budgeting, the occasional shopping addiction. But hey, I would rather focus on the positive than the negative – I wasted far too many years being negative, and it's now my time to shine. Pass the sequins, the glitter and the big earrings!

If you suspect you're neurodivergent (and even if you aren't), I want you to sit down and write a list of your own superpowers. Ask friends and family for help in pointing out those things they love about you. It's such an important part of the journey to recognise and embrace every part of you, especially when you've likely spent a whole lifetime trying to squash those traits. The added bonus of celebrating your full self is that you'll be modelling how to do it for your neurodivergent kids. It's win-win.

If you've recently been diagnosed, just know that your neurodivergence is not something to fix – it's something to celebrate. You, too, have unique strengths, or 'superpowers', that are part of who you are. Whether it's hyperfocus, creativity, problem-solving or simply seeing the world from a different perspective, these traits are valuable. Embrace them. Lean into what makes you different, because that's often where your greatest talents lie. The world needs neurosparkly minds like yours, and learning to honour your strengths will help you thrive. It's not about fitting into someone else's mould – it's about discovering and celebrating what makes *you* truly exceptional.

Q & A

Q: HOW DO I ACCOMMODATE MY CHILD'S SENSORY NEEDS AS WELL AS MY OWN WHEN WE ARE BOTH NEURODIVERGENT – PARTICULARLY IF THESE NEEDS CONFLICT?

A: Attending to the needs of everyone in your family, including – *especially* – your own can seem like an impossible task . . . particularly if you are both neurodivergent. No matter how much you love your child, when your sensory needs are different to theirs, this relationship can be really hard to navigate at times. After all, it's not easy to have a meltdown or a shutdown when you are also responsible for another little human.

You love loud music. They hate it.

You love tight hugs. They despise touch.

You love strong smells. They can't stand them.

It can be *so* hard trying to meet the needs of your child while also caring for yourself, but ultimately you also need to have your needs met (put your own oxygen mask on first and all of that). This is a good time to bring in all the things to support each of you.

Headphones for you that blast your favourite music and noise-cancelling headphones for them.

Tight hugs for you from someone else, or a big lap dog, who loves them (and compression singlets and weighted blankets to mimic it at other times) and light touch (or no touch) for them.

Scented candles and strong smellies for you in your room and neutral odours in theirs.

This is an opportune time to teach your child about others' needs and how they may differ from their own, and also a good time to teach them about consent. Don't try to hide your own needs or only cater to theirs – take this time to explain to them how you understand and respect their specific needs, and ask them to do the same for you.

It may mean you need to take more time out to decompress, getting up earlier in the day or going to bed later at night to ensure you have some alone time. It also means you may do things differently from other parents and – as long as it is not hurting anyone – this is okay. I tell parents that putting your child to bed earlier than normal to watch their favourite movie on an iPad in bed (even on a school night) to give you some time alone is totally fine. Often it is actually easier for our buzzing, noisy neurodivergent brains to fall asleep while watching something. I know I need to watch mindless TV (*The Kardashians*, anyone?) for my brain to truly switch off after a busy, stressful day, and our little people can be the exact same.

By learning to support your kids, you also learn to support your own needs. And who better to parent neurodivergent kids than neurodivergent parents?

Q: SHOULD I TELL MY WORKPLACE ABOUT MY NEW DIAGNOSIS?

A: Deciding whether to disclose your diagnosis at work is a personal choice that depends on your comfort level and the workplace environment. If you feel that sharing your diagnosis could lead to a better understanding of you, and accommodations that support you in doing your best work, then it may be worth considering. Many workplaces are becoming more aware of neurodivergence and are willing to make adjustments, such as flexible hours or sensory-friendly spaces. However, you don't have to disclose it if it doesn't feel safe or necessary. Ultimately, it's about what feels right for you – whether you decide to share it or keep it private, your neurodivergence is valid and valuable either way.

I recently had a woman come up to me after a conference and she quietly said, 'I am a psychologist who has recently been diagnosed autistic and ADHD, and I don't know whether I should tell my colleagues and clients.'

Here was a very smart, mature professional woman questioning whether she should share her diagnosis. I was genuinely intrigued, so we sat and spoke about it, and I encouraged her to unpack what it was she was worried about. She admitted she felt everyone would suddenly think she was an imposter and incapable of supporting neurodivergent people, because she was neurodivergent herself. She questioned whether her colleagues would look down on her and feel she wasn't their equal.

I assured her that she would be an incredible asset, because she truly understands the unique ways in which neurodivergent brains work. She would not just empathise – she would *get it* from lived experience. Having a therapist who shares your neurodivergent perspective means they are more likely to offer strategies and insights that genuinely resonate. They can also create a space where people feel seen and understood without having to constantly explain themselves. This connection can be so empowering, and I assured her *many* of my clients actively sought out neurodivergent professionals, and that she should not only announce it but embrace it and turn it into her speciality – her *superpower*!

As expected, her colleagues were not only fine (some also shared their own diagnoses), but her practice is *thriving* since she has changed her advertising strategies to loudly and proudly share her diagnosis and skills to support the neurodivergent community. And, of course, she is so much happier living as her authentic self.

Conclusion

If you've made it this far, congratulations! Just by reading this book, you've already taken a really important step to giving your child the support they need to thrive. Let's take a minute to appreciate and reflect on the massive journey we've taken together.

We've gotten our heads around the neurodivergent frameworks and language, and gained a few pro tips on how to begin parenting differently. We've explored the diagnosis pathways, acknowledging the huge range of traits that neurodivergence covers and how each neurodivergent child will display them in a unique way. We've gone back to the classroom for a biology lesson on the nervous system and equipped your toolbox for dealing with meltdowns, shutdowns and burnout.

You can try out many of the ideas for making family life more neurodivergent friendly quickly and easily, to get a sense of what will work for you and your child. When it comes to schooling, you've got all the options at your fingertips for accommodating your child's needs, whether that ends up being within the system or from home. Your child's mental wellbeing must remain a top priority, and you've got plenty of advice on hand for supporting this yourself or choosing from a range of professional support options. For puberty and that transition to adulthood, it's all about communication and empowering your child to find their own pathways to self-regulation and compassion. And for some of you, there'll be the extra journey of an adult diagnosis, for yourself and your partner, with all of the epiphanies that can bring.

I think you'll agree that all of this is a lot! A lot of information, a lot of feelings to manage, and a lot to process when it comes to applying this advice to your child. Be kind to yourself, and remember, you can revisit any chapter whenever you need to refresh on a particular topic.

My main wish for you is that reading this book has given you hope for the future, and you feel excited to not only better understand neurodivergence but also fully embrace it for the incredible gift it is – for your child and everyone in their orbit. Imagine how boring the world would be if all brains thought the same. We would be like bland robots with no rainbows or glitter!

I hope you walk away empowered, with a new strength to face the world and realise it's not your child – or you – that needs to change but the world around you. As Chloé's famous jacket says, 'fix the system, not me'. And by supporting your child to be their authentic self, you can help make that change.

As each day passes in the life of our family, we find a beautiful rhythm in the everyday moments – one that's built on love, acceptance, understanding and growth. It's present in the way each family member supports one another through challenges, celebrates small victories and embraces what makes them unique. Each person is accepted for exactly who they are, quirks and all. The journey isn't always easy, but it's filled with love, laughter, creativity and the deep bonds that come from navigating the world together. This family knows it's not about fitting the mould, but about discovering and honouring each person's needs, strengths and individuality. Oh, and taking the piss out of each other constantly – but all in good spirits! At the end of the day, it's this unwavering love, patience and joy in the little things that makes the home a safe and empowering space where everyone is free to be exactly who they are – neurosparkly or not – and that is truly something to cherish.

Acknowledgements

I have been writing since I was a little girl. I still have books at home I self-published and printed out as a young child, dreaming of one day being a *real* author. When I was asked in primary school what I wanted to be when I grew up, I simply answered 'author'. I had no idea what I would write, I just knew I *needed* to write. A few years ago, I made the decision I would be a published author by the age of 50 . . . and just left it to the universe to provide.

When I received an email from Alexandra Payne at Murdoch Books wanting to discuss me writing a book on parenting neuro-divergent kids, I actually googled her to see if she was real. Alex has been my biggest supporter and kept her faith in me even when I lost faith in myself. Alex, thank you for checking in when I went quiet, for encouraging me to keep writing when I didn't think I had any more words in me, and for having patience every time I missed a deadline (there were *many*!).

Thank you to my editorial manager, Julie Mazur Tribe, who popped in and out like a fairy godmother, checking on me and my team, encouraging me and confirming I was on the right path to creating a wonderful book.

And to the gorgeous Nikki Lusk, my editor, thank you for helping me to create magic.

Thank you to everyone at Murdoch Books who saw something in me when I couldn't see it in myself, for all the love and support you have given me, and especially for making my dream of being a published author come true.

To my children, thank you for being my greatest teachers, my most honest critics and the reason I get out of bed each day. Thank you for providing endless material for this book – you have taught me more than any research paper or degree ever could. Your unique ways of seeing the world have made mine so much bigger, and you have shown me that neurodivergence is a gift and a superpower, even if it comes with the occasional meltdown.

A huge shout-out to the neurodivergent community – parents, kids, educators, therapists and friends who generously shared their stories, wisdom and sometimes their moments of chaos and despair. This book is nothing without you. Thank you for reminding me daily why I do what I do. To all my beautiful clients, thank you for being so wonderfully weird and creative and quirky (in the best possible way). Your stories gave this book heart, and your resilience gave it hope. I love you all and am so thankful for the trust you put in me.

Thank you to my neurosparkly friends Madeleine and Sharon, who read snippets of my book and gave me feedback and encouragement. I am so grateful to have found you. You came into my life right when I needed you and are the most wonderful cheerleaders a girl could ask for.

To my beautiful mum, who passed away in 2020, I can only imagine how proud you would be of this book. I love and miss you more than you could ever know. Thank you for always encouraging me to write as a child, and for always encouraging my children to be themselves. There is not a day that goes by that I don't want to call you to tell you my news – and I know this book news would have been so exciting for you.

To my lifelong partner and best friend in the whole wide world, Ronnie, thank you for being brave enough to share your diagnosis story – I couldn't be prouder of you. Thank you for the morning cups of coffee, for topping up my prosecco glass in the evening, for sitting on the couch until well after midnight while I read and re-read my chapters to you. For someone who is dyslexic, you sure have a gift with words. Thank you for not allowing me to give up when I would dramatically shut my computer saying, 'I can't do this anymore!'.

Finally, thank you, dear reader, for having the courage to pick up this book. Those of us who are willing to *parent differently* will help create an environment in which our children can thrive. Thank you for walking with me.

Resources

Here are some organisations and other resources that may support you and your child in discovering more about neurodivergence and how to connect with services and others in the neurodivergent community.

Obviously, for the neurodivergent teens and young adults in your life I must recommend the book by the one and only Chloé Hayden, *Different, Not Less* (Murdoch Books, 2022). Chloé's podcast, *Boldly Me*, also has some great interviews with other neurodivergent superstars.

I have a business with my girlfriend Sharon Witt, a renowned author and educator, where we bring our combined expertise and lived experience as neurodivergent women to create meaningful change. Through our business and podcast *Two Neurosparkly Gals*, we are committed to building spaces where neurodivergent individuals feel understood, supported and empowered on their unique journeys. With a shared mission to raise awareness, we offer practical guidance to help workplaces and educational settings become more neuro-affirming, fostering inclusivity and understanding. By sharing authentic stories and actionable insights, we inspire others to embrace the strengths of neurodiversity, ultimately empowering individuals and communities to thrive together. You can find all the details of our conferences, other talks, panels and useful resources at twoneurosparklygals.com

*Organisations marked with ** offer international support.*

Australia

ADHD

ADDults with ADHD
Authoritative information, publications and services to support adults with ADHD and their families and friends. Events include quarterly ADHD afternoons led by speakers and a chance to meet and chat with others.
adultadhd.org.au

ADHD Australia
Support groups, research and a newsletter sharing the latest information and resources for ADHD folk and their families.
adhdaustralia.org.au

Autism

Amaze
Information and resources for autistic people and their families and supporters, including workshops, online resources and an autism helpline via phone, email or live chat.
amaze.org.au • Helpline: 1300 308 699

Aspect
Australia's largest autism-specific service provider, working in partnership with autistic people of all ages and their families.
aspect.org.au

Autism Advisory and Support Service
Offering autistic people, their families and carers a holistic approach to service delivery.
aass.org.au

Autism Awareness Australia
Empowering autism families with information, education, awareness and advocacy for inclusion.
autismawareness.com.au

Autism Friendly Charter

A directory of businesses, organisations and agencies that have completed specific inclusion and accessibility training developed in collaboration with the autistic community.
autismfriendlycharter.org.au

Happy Families

Neurodiversity-affirming course for parents and carers of autistic children.
happyfamilies.com.au

I CAN Network

Professional development workshops and campaigns to increase autism understanding.
icannetwork.online

Positive Partnerships

Workshops, webinars and online modules for parents, carers and school staff to strengthen their capacity to support the autistic kids in their lives.
positivepartnerships.com.au

Yellow Ladybugs

Support and informal events for autistic girls and gender-diverse individuals between the ages of five and sixteen.
yellowladybugs.com.au

Bipolar disorder

Bipolar Australia

Education and resources for bipolar people and their families, friends and carers.
bipolaraustralia.org.au

Bullying

eSafety Commissioner (Australian Government)

Education guides and webinars for parents to learn more about bullying, with a pathway to report cyberbullying.
esafety.gov.au

Carers

Carer Gateway

Emotional and practical services and support for carers.
carergateway.gov.au

Carers Australia

Information and support for carers.
carersaustralia.com.au

Complex trauma
Australian Childhood Foundation
Therapeutic trauma care for children traumatised by abuse, neglect and family violence.
childhood.org.au

Blue Knot
Phone counselling, resources and workshops for adults affected by childhood trauma and abuse. Also educates and trains people to support survivors.
blueknot.org.au • Helpline and Redress Support Service: 1300 657 380

Disability support
**Hidden Disabilities Sunflower
The sunflower lanyard is a simple tool for voluntarily sharing that you have a hidden disability and might need extra help, understanding or just more time.
hdsunflower.com

Down syndrome
Down Syndrome Australia
Supports and services for people with Down syndrome, their families and supporters.
downsyndrome.org.au

Dyslexia, Dyspraxia and Dyscalculia
Australian Dyslexia Association
Guidance for parents to identify dyslexia in their children and find support, particularly in educational services.
dyslexiaassociation.org.au

Developmental Coordination Disorder Australia Inc.
Awareness-raising, education and support for kids with developmental coordination disorder, or dyspraxia, and their families.
dcdaustralia.org.au

Auspeld
Representing and supporting children with specific learning disorders across Australia.
auspeld.org.au

Eating disorders
Butterfly Foundation
Support for all people affected by eating disorders and negative body image – the person with the illness, their family and their friends.
butterfly.org.au

Embrace Kids

Resources for families, educators and community sports clubs to promote a world where young people are free from feelings of pressure, judgement and shame about their bodies.
theembracehub.com

General mental health

Beyond Blue

Information and support to help everyone in Australia achieve their best possible mental health.
beyondblue.org.au • 1300 224 636

Black Dog Institute

A transnational research institute that aims to reduce the incidence of mental illness and the stigma around it, to actively reduce suicide rates and empower everyone to live the most mentally healthy lives possible.
blackdoginstitute.org.au

Embrace Multicultural Mental Health

Mental health and suicide prevention services for people from culturally and linguistically diverse backgrounds.
embracementalhealth.org.au

Headspace

The National Youth Mental Health Foundation, providing early intervention mental health services to young people aged 12–25, along with assistance in promoting the wellbeing of young people.
headspace.org.au

Kids Helpline

Australia's only free, private and confidential 24/7 phone and online counselling service for young people between the ages of 5 and 25.
kidshelpline.com.au • 1800 551 800

Lifeline

National 24-hour crisis support and suicide prevention services.
lifeline.org.au • 13 11 14

The Resilience Project

Emotionally engaging programs for schools, sports clubs and businesses, providing practical, evidence-based mental health strategies to build resilience and happiness.
theresilienceproject.com.au

LGBTQIA+

Minus18

LGBTQIA+ resources, workplace training, school workshops and events for youth across Australia.
minus18.org.au

Parents of Gender Diverse Children
Direct support for parents of trans or gender diverse kids.
pgdc.org.au

Switchboard
Peer-driven support and resources for members of the LGBTQIA+ community, their families, allies and the community.
switchboard.org.au

Transcend Australia
Family and peer support, education, resources and advocacy programs for trans, gender-diverse and non-binary children and young people.
transcend.org.au

Mindfulness

**Cosmic Kids
Yoga and mindfulness for kids aged three to eight.
cosmickids.com

Soundwalks (ABC Kids Listen)
Guided relaxation exercises for kids.
abc.net.au/kidslisten/programs/soundwalks

OCD

So OCD
Education, resources and support for people with OCD and their families.
soocd.com.au

Puberty

Planet Puberty
Guidance for parents of kids with intellectual disability and autism for their child's journey through puberty.
planetpuberty.org.au

School

Euka Future Learning
Resources, information and curriculums for homeschooling parents.
euka.edu.au

My HomeSchool
Guidance and curriculums for homeschooling parents.
myhomeschool.com

Student Wellbeing Hub
Supporting physical, mental and emotional wellbeing in schools.
studentwellbeinghub.edu.au

Sex education

SECCA
Resources, education and support for people with disability to learn about relationships, sexuality and sexual health.
secca.org.au

Sexual assault

1800RESPECT
Free and confidential support 24 hours a day, every day, for sexual assault, domestic and family violence counselling, information and referrals.
1800respect.org.au • 1800 737 732

Bravehearts
Counselling and education for children and young people as well as parental support, training and research to combat issues associated with child sexual assault.
bravehearts.org.au • 1800 272 831

Social connections

Wondiverse
Neuroinclusive education, resources and social connections.
wondiverse.com.au

Tourette syndrome

Tourette Syndrome Association of Australia Inc.
Support for people with Tourette syndrome and their families.
tourette.org.au

IRELAND/UNITED KINGDOM

ADHD

ADHD Foundation
Services, resources and events for autism, ADHD, dyslexia, dyspraxia, dyscalculia and Tourette syndrome.
adhdfoundation.org.uk

ADHD Ireland
Resources, support, events, social outings and a dedicated phone and email hotline for people with ADHD and their families and carers.
adhdireland.ie • 01 874 8349

ADHD UK
Provides an online guide to support groups that span across the United Kingdom.
adhduk.co.uk

Autism

As I Am
An autistic-led charity that offers training, education, support and resources.
asiam.ie

AUsome Training
A community organisation run by autistic people that offers in-person and online courses to address the inaccurate portrayal of autism. Also the home of AUsome Cork, an annual conference featuring autistic advocates who educate the general public about the needs of autistic people.
ausometraining.com

Autistic Inclusive Meets (AIM)
A not-for-profit autistic advocacy organisation created by autistic people that focuses on promoting autism acceptance, protesting against laws that harm autistic people and connecting the autistic community. Hosts weekly meet-ups and events for the autistic community, both in person and online.
autisticinclusivemeets.org

National Autistic Society
Support, guidance, diagnostic services, professional development, and education and employment opportunities for autistic people.
autism.org.uk

Bipolar disorder

Aware
Support, education and information for Irish people impacted by bipolar disorder and their families and caregivers.
aware.ie

Bipolar UK
Support groups for people affected by bipolar, as well as their families, loved ones and friends.
bipolaruk.org

Bullying

National Bullying Helpline
Guidance and advice for parents about bullying.
nationalbullyinghelpline.co.uk • 0300 323 0169

Tackle Bullying
National website to counter bullying and cyberbullying in Ireland for young people, parents and teachers.
tacklebullying.ie

Carers

Carers UK
Help and advice for carers and professionals.
carersuk.org

Family Carers Ireland
Support that promotes the health, wellbeing and quality of life for family carers and those for whom they care.
familycarers.ie

Down syndrome

Down's Syndrome Association
Education, helpline and advocacy for people with Down syndrome and their families.
downs-syndrome.org.uk

Down Syndrome Ireland
Support for people with Down syndrome, their families and professionals.
downsyndrome.ie

Dyslexia, Dyspraxia and Dyscalculia

British Dyslexia Association
Resources and support for people with dyslexia and dyscalculia.
bdadyslexia.org.uk

Dyslexia Ireland
Information, support and advocacy for people affected by dyslexia and dyscalculia.
dyslexia.ie

Dyspraxia/DCD Ireland
Supports and services for young people and adults with dyspraxia/DCD and their families and supporters.
dyspraxia.ie

The Brain Charity
Practical and emotional support for people living with dyspraxia all over the United Kingdom.
thebraincharity.org.uk

Eating disorders

Beat Eating Disorders
Information, advice and a supportive online community for those affected by eating disorders. They have helplines in England, Scotland, Wales and Northern Ireland that run 365 days per year.
beateatingdisorders.org.uk

Eating Disorders Association NI
Free and confidential support for anyone living with an eating disorder, for their family, friends and carers, and for professionals working with eating disorders.
eatingdisordersni.co.uk

General mental health
Childline
Free counselling for children and young people with any issue they may be confronting.
childline.org.uk • 0800 1111

Mind
Advice and support to empower anyone experiencing a mental health problem.
mind.org.uk • 0300 123 3393

National Suicide Prevention Helpline
A supportive listening service for anyone with thoughts of suicide.
nsphuk.org • 0800 689 5652

Samaritans
Free, confidential mental health support via phone or email.
samaritans.org • 116 123

SANEline
National out-of-hours helpline for mental health support.
sane.org.uk • 0300 304 7000

Shout
Free, confidential mental health support 24/7 via text.
giveusashout.org • Text 'shout' to 85258

LGBTQIA+
AKT
Support for LGBTQIA+ young people aged 16–25 who are facing or experiencing homelessness or living in a hostile environment, helping them to stay safe in crisis situations, find emergency accommodation, access specialist support and develop skills and life goals.
akt.org.uk • 020 7831 6562

LGBT Ireland
Resources and local peer-support groups for LGBTQIA+ people and their families, also offering online chat functions and two helplines, one for general LGBTQIA+ and one for transgender family support.
lgbt.ie • 1800 929 539 (LGBT Support Line) • 01 907 3707 (Transgender Family Support Line)

Mermaids

Resources and support for trans, non-binary and gender-questioning children and young people, and the important people in their lives, including a helpline and parents group.
mermaidsuk.org.uk • 080 8801 0400

Switchboard

Peer-driven support and resources for LGBTQIA+ people, their families, allies and the community.
switchboard.lgbt • 0300 330 0630

OCD

OCD Ireland

Support groups and information for people with OCD and their families.
ocdireland.org

OCD UK

Advice, information and support services for those affected by OCD.
ocduk.org

Sex education

Fumble

Free digital sex education resources and support for young people and their parents.
fumble.org.uk

Sexual assault

Safeline

Free, specialist, best-practice services for adults and children affected by or at risk of sexual violence.
safeline.org.uk • 01926 402 498

The Survivors Trust

Counselling, therapeutic and support services for victims of rape, sexual violence and sexual abuse, including free, confidential helpline and live chat services.
thesurvivorstrust.org • 0808 801 0818

Tourette syndrome

Tourettes Action

Support and resources for people in the United Kingdom with Tourette syndrome and their families.
tourettes-action.org.uk

Tourette's Support NI

Support meetings, training services, awareness and education campaigns and activities for children with Tourette syndrome and their families.
tourettessupportni.org

CANADA/UNITED STATES OF AMERICA

ADHD

**ADDitude

A quarterly magazine and online resource for people living with ADHD, providing access to evidence-based information, free webinars, an online community and more.
additudemag.com

CHADD

Education, advocacy and support for children and adults living with ADHD and their families, as well as teachers and healthcare professionals.
chadd.org • 866 200 8098

Autism

**Autistic Women & Nonbinary Network (AWN)

An autistic-led organisation that provides community, support and resources for autistic women, girls, nonbinary people and all others of marginalised genders. They also provide support for minority groups, such as autistic LGBTQIA+ people and autistic people of colour. AWN provides opportunities to connect the autistic community through networking, educational and social gatherings, autism acceptance events, book readings and autistic pride picnics.
awnnetwork.org

Autistics for Autistics (A4A) Ontario

Support to improve rights and opportunities for autistic Canadian people, especially in the areas of school inclusion, employment, housing and access to medical care.
a4aontario.com

Autistics United Canada

A disability rights organisation created by autistic people that focuses on building a community of autistic people while fostering autistic identity and pride. The Vancouver chapter has a mobile neurodiversity library with books about autism acceptance as well as fidget gadgets for autistic people.
autisticsunitedca.org

**Nonspeaking CommUnity Consortium

A not-for-profit organisation founded by nonspeaking autistic and other neurodivergent nonspeaking people and allies that promotes communication access and choice.

de-de.facebook.com/groups/nonspeakingcommunity/

Bipolar disorder

**International Bipolar Foundation

Education, resources and supportive connection for all who are touched by bipolar disorder.

ibpf.org

Bullying

Bullying Canada

Wrap-around mental health service for bullied youth.

bullyingcanada.ca

Stop Bullying

Resources for US-based parents about bullying and cyberbullying.

stopbullying.gov

Down syndrome

Canadian Down Syndrome Society (CDSS)

Resources and support for the Down syndrome community.

cdss.ca

National Down Syndrome Society

Resources, support and advocacy for US-based people with Down syndrome and their families.

ndss.org

Dyslexia, dyspraxia and dyscalculia

CanChild

Resources for Canadian parents and educators about children with dyspraxia/DCD.

canchild.ca

**Dyscalculia.org

Educational resources and support group for people with dyscalculia.

dyscalculia.org

Dyslexia Canada

Resources and peer support program for parents and caregivers of children with dyslexia.

dyslexiacanada.org

Dyspraxia Foundation USA
Raising awareness, educating and supporting those living with dyspraxia, their parents and their families.
dyspraxiausa.org

Learning Disabilities Association of America
Resources, advocacy and localised support for people with learning disabilities, their families and educators.
ldaamerica.org

Eating disorders
National Eating Disorders Association (NEDA)
Support for people affected by eating disorders, including treatment options, support groups, events and helplines in the form of online chat, call and text.
nationaleatingdisorders.org • 800 931 2237

General mental health
988 Suicide & Crisis Lifeline
Free, 24/7 and confidential support for people in distress, as well as prevention and crisis resources, and best practices for professionals.
988lifeline.org • 988

TheHopeLine
Resources for people struggling with poor mental health, including suicide and mental health resources, email mentors, prayer, weekly personalised emails and live chat service.
thehopeline.com

LGBTQIA+
Families in TRANSition
Educational group for Canadian parents and caregivers of transgender, nonbinary or gender-questioning youth aged five to seventeen.
ok2bme.ca/services/fit/

**GLAAD
Empowers the LGBTQIA+ community by sharing their stories, holding the media accountable for the words and images they present, and helping grassroots organisations communicate effectively.
glaad.org

**The Trevor Project
Suicide prevention support for lesbian, gay, bisexual, transgender, queer and questioning youth. The toll-free Trevor Lifeline is a confidential service that offers trained counsellors, as well as resources, public education and research.
thetrevorproject.org • 866 488 7386

TransParent

Connections and resources for US-based parents and caregivers navigating the complex issues faced by their gender-expansive children of any age.
transparentusa.org

OCD

**International OCD Foundation

Educational resources, community events and programs for people with OCD.
iocdf.org

Sexual assault

RAINN

Anti-sexual violence services, public education, public policy, consulting services and a national hotline in partnership with more than 1000 local sexual assault service providers across the United States, offering online live chat and telephone helplines.
rainn.org • 800-656-4673

Tourette syndrome

Tourette Canada

Education, advocacy and community outreach for children, adults and families living with Tourette syndrome.
tourette.ca

Tourette Association of America

Resources and support groups for people with Tourette syndrome and their families.
tourette.org

Notes

Chapter 1: Parenting the neurosparkly way

The word neurodiversity *recognises and embraces*: M. Botha, R. Chapman, M. Giwa Onaiwu et al., 'The neurodiversity concept was developed collectively: An overdue correction on the origins of neurodiversity theory', *Autism*, vol. 28, no. 6, pp. 1591–1954, doi.org/10.1177/13623613241237871

Neurodivergence *refers to*: Kassiane Asusamasu came up with the word 'neurodivergence' in the early 2000s: K. Asusamasu, 'PSA from the actual coiner of "neurodivergent"', 1 July 2021, brightlotusmoon.tumblr.com/post/655527684253892608/psa-from-the-actual-coiner-of-neurodivergent

Autism, which describes differences: Reframing Autism, 'What is autism?', reframingautism.org.au/about-autism/

ADHD, or attention deficit hyperactivity disorder: ADDitude editors, 'What is ADHD?' ADDitude, 26 September 2019, additudemag.com/what-is-adhd-symptoms-causes-treatments/

Bipolar disorder, which can be seen: S. Collier, 'Bipolar disorder', Harvard Health Publishing, 8 March 2023, health.harvard.edu/a_to_z/bipolar-disorder-manic-depressive-illness-or-manic-depression-a-to-z

Down syndrome, where a person is born: Down Syndrome Australia, 'What is Down syndrome?', downsyndrome.org.au/about-down-syndrome/what-is-down-syndrome/

Dyslexia involves difficulties: M. Hebert, D. Kearns, J.B. Hayes et al., 'Why children with dyslexia struggle with writing and how to help them', *Language, Speech, and Hearing Services in Schools*, vol. 49, no. 4, October 2018, pp. 843–863.

Dyspraxia refers to a brain's inability: NHS, 'Developmental co-ordination disorder (dyspraxia) in children', 8 March 2023, nhs.uk/conditions/developmental-coordination-disorder-dyspraxia/

Dyscalculia looks like: Dyslexia – SPELD Foundation, 'What is Dyscalculia?', dsf.net.au/learning-difficulties/dyscalculia/what-is-dyscalculia

OCD, or obsessive compulsive disorder: National Institute of Mental Health, 'Obsessive-Compulsive Disorder: when unwanted thoughts or repetitive behaviors take over', nimh.nih.gov/health/publications/obsessive-compulsive-disorder-when-unwanted-thoughts-or-repetitive-behaviors-take-over

Tourette syndrome is characterised: Tourettes action, 'What is Tourette Syndrome?', tourettes-action.org.uk/67-what-is-ts.html

more than 50 per cent co-occurrence of Tourette Syndrome and ADHD: M.E. Hirschtritt, P.C. Lee, D.L. Pauls et al., 'Lifetime prevalence, age of risk, and etiology of comorbid psychiatric disorders in Tourette syndrome', *JAMA Psychiatry*, vol. 72, no. 4, April 2015, pp. 325–333, ncbi.nlm.nih.gov/pmc/articles/PMC4446055/

50–70 per cent of autistic people also have ADHD: C. Hours, C. Recasens, J-M. Baleyte, 'ASD and ADHD comorbidity: what are we talking about?', *Front Psychiatry*, eCollection, 28 February 2022, pubmed.ncbi.nlm.nih.gov/35295773/

many of us will mask: B. Radulski, 'What are "masking" and "camouflaging" in the context of autism and ADHD?', *The Conversation*, 9 January 2023, theconversation.com/what-are-masking-and-camouflaging-in-the-context-of-autism-and-adhd-193446

Neurodivergent people are more likely ... to identify as gender-diverse: J.F. Strang, L. Kenworthy, A. Dominska et al., 'Increased gender variance in autism spectrum disorders and attention deficit hyperactivity disorder', *Archives of Sexual Behavior*, vol. 43, no. 8, November 2014, pp. 1525–1533, pubmed.ncbi.nlm.nih.gov/24619651/

it comes from Hans Asperger: S. Baron-Cohen, 'The truth about Hans Asperger's Nazi collusion', 8 May 2018, nature.com/articles/d41586-018-05112-1

a growing number of researchers: R. Nuwer, 'Finding strengths in autism', *The Transmitter*, 12 May 2021, thetransmitter.org/spectrum/finding-strengths-in-autism/

Neuropsychologist Isabelle Soulieres says: Nuwer, 'Finding strengths in autism'.

Kate Cooper, a research fellow: Nuwer, 'Finding strengths in autism'.

The online Urban Dictionary.com describes an 'autism mom': Urban Dictionary, 'autism mom', 12 April 2023, urbandictionary.com/define.php?term=autism%20mom

An autism mum sees themselves: J. Meadows, 'The autism mom: why is she like that?', *Medium*, 15 May 2021, jessemeadows.medium.com/the-autism-mom-why-is-she-like-that-c2f8cb2572bf

many autistic people may feel the emotions of others: I. Shalev, V. Warrier, D.M. Greenberg et al., 'Reexamining empathy in autism: empathic disequilibrium as a novel predictor of autism diagnosis and autism traits', *Autism Research*, vol. 15, no. 10, October 2022, pp. 1917–1928, ncbi.nlm.nih.gov/pmc/articles/PMC9804307/

Chapter 2: Diagnosis (aka discovery!)

girls' traits being treated differently: K. Lundin, S. Mahdi, J. Isaksson et al., 'Functional gender differences in autism: an international, multidisciplinary expert survery using the International Classification of Functioning, Disability, and Health model', *Autism*, vol. 25, no. 4, 2021, pp. 1020–1035, journals.sagepub.com/doi/full/10.1177/1362361320975311

racial bias can make a diagnosis more difficult: D. Straiton and A. Sridhar, 'Short report: call to action for autism clinicians in response to anti-Black racism', *Autism*, vol. 26, no. 4, 2022, pp. 988–994, journals.sagepub.com/doi/full/10.1177/13623613211043643

autistic children are more likely to not identify with the sex they were assigned at birth: V. Warrier, D.M. Greenberg, E. Weir et al., 'Elevated rates of autism, other neurodevelopmental and psychiatric diagnoses, and autistic traits in transgender and gender-diverse individuals', *Nature Communications*, vol. 11, no. 1, p. 3959, pubmed.ncbi.nlm.nih.gov/32770077/

Girls and women are commonly misdiagnosed: C. Gesi, G. Migliarese, S. Torriero et al., 'Gender differences in misdiagnosis and delayed diagnosis among adults with Autism Spectrum Disorder with no language or intellectual disability', *Brain Sciences*, vol. 11, no. 7, July 2021, p. 912, ncbi.nlm.nih.gov/pmc/articles/PMC8306851/

ADHD can present in kids as: 'ADHD symptoms in children', *ADDitude*, additudemag.com/category/adhd-add/adhd-in-children/add-symptoms/

Chapter 3: Neurosparkly nervous systems

rocking and gentle movement can help calm a baby's nervous system: C. Bergland, 'The neuroscience of calming a baby', *Psychology Today*, 22 April 2013, psychologytoday.com/au/blog/the-athletes-way/201304/the-neuroscience-calming-baby

the nervous system is the body's communication network: 'Nervous system', *healthdirect*, healthdirect.gov.au/nervous-system

the sympathetic nervous system will prime the body: 'What is the fight, flight, freeze or fawn response?', Cleveland Clinic, 22 July 2024, health.clevelandclinic.org/what-happens-to-your-body-during-the-fight-or-flight-response

Anxiety is also common in neurodivergent people: O.T. Leyfer, S.E. Folstein, S. Bacalman et al., 'Comorbid psychiatric disorders in children with autism: interview development and rates of disorders', *Journal of Autism and Development Disorders*, vol. 36, no. 7, October 2006, pp. 849–861, pubmed.ncbi.nlm.nih.gov/16845581/; S.L. Gair, H.R. Brown, S. Kang et al., 'Early development of comorbidity between symptoms of ADHD and anxiety', *Research on Child and Adolescent Psychopathology*, vol. 49, no. 3, March 2021, pp. 311–323, ncbi.nlm.nih.gov/pmc/articles/PMC7878348/

deep breathing exercises can help activate the parasympathetic nervous system: 'Proper breathing brings better health', *Scientific American*, 15 January 2019, scientificamerican.com/article/proper-breathing-brings-better-health/

spending time in nature has been linked: 'A 20-minute nature break relieves stress', Harvard Health Publishing, 1 July 2019, health.harvard.edu/mind-and-mood/a-20-minute-nature-break-relieves-stress

Stimming can be a natural way to release built-up energy and regain a sense of calm: S.K. Kapp, R. Steward, L. Crane et al., '"People should be allowed to do what they like": autistic adults' views and experiences of stimming', *Autism*, vol. 23, no. 7, 2019, pp. 1782–1792, journals.sagepub.com/doi/full/10.1177/1362361319829628

EMDR ... and somatic experiencing use similar rhythmic or repetitive movements: R. Landin-Romero, A. Moreno-Alcazar, M. Pagani et al., 'How does Eye Movement Desensitization and Reprocessing Therapy work? A systematic review on suggested mechanisms of action', *Frontiers in Psychology*, vol. 9, 2018, p. 1395, ncbi.nlm.nih.gov/pmc/articles/PMC6106867/; P. Payne, P.A. Levine and M.A. Crane-Godreau, 'Somatic experiencing: using interoception and proprioception as core elements of trauma therapy', *Frontiers in Psychology*, vol. 6, 2015, p. 93, ncbi.nlm.nih.gov/pmc/articles/PMC4316402/

a meltdown is an intense response: 'Meltdowns: a guide for all audiences', National Autistic Society, autism.org.uk/advice-and-guidance/topics/behaviour/meltdowns/all-audiences; L. Batten, 'Strategies to manage and prevent ADHD-related meltdowns', The Mini ADHD Coach, 21 January 2022, theminiadhdcoach.com/living-with-adhd/adhd-meltdown

at *a higher risk of burnout*: G. Brattberg, 'PTSD and ADHD: underlying factors in many cases of burnout', *Stress & Health*, vol. 22, no. 5, December 2006, pp. 305–313, onlinelibrary.wiley.com/doi/abs/10.1002/smi.1112

a totally distinct condition: R.B. Wheeler, 'Adult ADHD and burnout', 14 July 2022, WebMD, webmd.com/add-adhd/adult-adhd-burnout; D.M. Raymaker, A.R. Teo, N.A. Steckler et al., '"Having all of your internal resources exhausted beyond measure and being left with no clean-up crew": defining autistic burnout', *Autism Adulthood*, vol. 2, no. 2, 1 June 2020, pp. 132–143, pubmed.ncbi.nlm.nih.gov/32851204/

Most of the research on neurodivergent burnout comes from autism: S. West, 'Masking ADHD, autism, and dyslexia: burnout in neurodivergent individuals', presentation, Nordic Network on Disability Research Conference, May 2023, researchgate.net/publication/370764983_Masking_ADHD_Autism_and_Dyslexia_Burnout_in_Neurodivergent_Individuals_Summer_West

Neurodivergent burnout ... can look like: '"Having all of your internal resources exhausted beyond measure and being left with no clean-up crew"'; H. Edgar, 'Supporting children through autistic burnout (parent/carer guide)', Autistic Realms, 5 December 2022, autisticrealms. com/post/supporting-children-through-autistic-burnout-parents-guide

Chapter 4: Family life

correlation between gastrointestinal problems and neurodivergence: B. Donaghy, D. Moore and J. Green, 'Co-occurring physical health challenges in neurodivergent children and young people: a topical review and recommendation', *Child Care in Practice*, vol. 29, no. 1, 2023, pp. 3–21, tandfonline.com/doi/full/10.1080/13575279.2022.2149471#d1e190

Animals can help develop social, sensory and communication skills: 'The power of pets: health benefits of human–animal interactions', National Institutes of Health, February 2018, newsinhealth.nih.gov/2018/02/power-pets

practising [gratitude] every day: 'Practicing gratitude: ways to improve positivity', National Institutes of Health, March 2019, newsinhealth.nih. gov/2019/03/practicing-gratitude

Chapter 5: School

neurotypical peers typically struggle to understand the way our kids interact and communicate: 'Milton's "double empathy problem": a summary for non-academics', Reframing Autism, reframingautism.org.au/miltons-double-empathy-problem-a-summary-for-non-academics/

our neurodivergent kids are particularly susceptible to bullying: P.D. Lin and V. Eapen, 'Kids on the autism spectrum experience more bullying. Schools can do something about it', *The Conversation*, 9 June 2022, theconversation.com/kids-on-the-autism-spectrum-experience-more-bullying-schools-can-do-something-about-it-184385

school refusal ... is very common in neurodivergent kids: J.E. Granieri, H.E. Morton, R.G. Romanczyk et al., 'Profiles of school refusal among neurodivergent youth', *European Education*, vol. 55, no. 3–4, 2023, pp. 186–201, tandfonline.com/doi/full/10.1080/10564934.2023.2251013

real physical symptoms from mental health challenges: 'Recognising and easing the physical symptoms of anxiety', Harvard Health Publishing, 29 July 2024, health.harvard.edu/mind-and-mood/recognizing-and-easing-the-physical-symptoms-of-anxiety

Chapter 6: Mental wellbeing

38 per cent of Australian autistic people experience anxiety and depression: A.L. Richdale, A. Haschek, L.P. Lawson et al., 'Supporting mental health: what young Australian autistic adults tell us', La Trobe University, Melbourne, doi.org/10.26181/5fdc10c56879a *autistic women are thirteen times more likely*: P. Jachyra, J. Rodgers, S. Cassidy, 'Autistic people are six times more likely to attempt suicide – poor mental health support may be to blame', *The Conversation*, 1 April 2022, theconversation.com/autistic-people-are-six-times-more-likely-to-attempt-suicide-poor-mental-health-support-may-be-to-blame-180266

People with ADHD commonly suffer from: Royal College of Psychiatrists, 'ADHD in adults', rcpsych.ac.uk/mental-health/mental-illnesses-and-mental-health-problems/adhd-in-adults

At least half of people with Down syndrome will face: National Down Syndrome Society, 'Mental health & Down syndrome', ndss.org/resources/mental-health-down-syndrome

neuro-affirming therapy is an approach: J. Barbaro, 'Neuroaffirming care values the strengths and differences of autistic people, those with ADHD or other profiles. Here's how', *The Conversation*, 8 May 2024, theconversation.com/neuroaffirming-care-values-the-strengths-and-differences-of-autistic-people-those-with-adhd-or-other-profiles-heres-how-227449

'you start pretty much from scratch when you work with an autistic child': P. Chance, 'A conversation with Ivar Lovaas about self-mutilating children and how their parents make it worse', *Psychology Today*, January 1974, republished on 5 July 2021 at just1voice.com/advocacy/ole-ivar-lovaas-interview-about-autism

40 hours a week: see, for example: Steps to Progress, 'Does my child really need 40 hours a week of ABA therapy?' 7 July 2023, stepstoprogress.com/blog/aba-therapy/does-my-child-need-40-hours/

autistic adults who mask are more prone: B. Radulski, 'What are "masking" and "camouflaging" in the context of autism and ADHD?' *The Conversation*, 9 January 2023, theconversation.com/what-are-masking-and-camouflaging-in-the-context-of-autism-and-adhd-193446

strong correlation between undergoing ABA and experiencing PTSD: H. Kupferstein, 'Evidence of increased PTSD symptoms in autistics exposed to applied behavior analysis', *Advances in Autism*, vol. 4, no. 3, January 2018, pp. 19–29, researchgate.net/publication/322239353_Evidence_of_increased_PTSD_symptoms_in_autistics_exposed_to_applied_behavior_analysis

Many neurodivergent adults who underwent ABA therapy as children: 'ABA horror stories are far too common', NeuroClastic, 17 August 2021, neuroclastic.com/aba-horror-stories-are-far-too-common/

Both ABA and gay conversion therapy: F. Fahrenheit, 'An open letter to the NYT: acknowledge the controversy surrounding ABA', NeuroClastic, 11 January 2020, neuroclastic.com/an-open-letter-to-the-nyt-acknowledge-the-controversy-surrounding-aba/

around 70 per cent of those with eating disorders: R. Juli, M.R. Juli, G. Juli et al., 'Eating disorders and psychiatric comorbidity', *Psychiatria Danubina*, vol. 35, supplement 2, October 2023, pp. 217–220.

Anorexia nervosa involves and other definitions in this paragraph: 'Eating disorders', National Institute of Mental Health, January 2024, nimh. nih.gov/health/topics/eating-disorders

20 to 35 per cent of women with anorexia: H. Westwood and K. Tchanturia, 'Autism spectrum disorder in anorexia nervosa: an updated literature review', *Current Psychiatry Reports*, vol. 19, no. 41, 2017, doi.org/ 10.1007/s11920-017-0791-9

People with ADHD, meanwhile, are more prone: J.R. Bleck, R.D. DeBate and R. Olivardia, 'The comorbidity of ADHD and eating disorders in a nationally representative sample', *Journal of Behavioral Health Services & Research*, vol. 42, no. 4, October 2015, pp. 437–451.

ARFID (avoidant/restrictive food intake disorder) is categorised: 'Eating disorders', National Institute of Mental Health, January 2024, nimh. nih.gov/health/topics/eating-disorders

ARFID frequently co-occurs with autism: A. Keski-Rahkonen and A. Ruusunen, 'Avoidant-restrictive food intake disorder and autism: epidemiology, etiology, complications, treatment, and outcome', *Current Opinions in Psychiatry*, vol. 36, no. 6, 1 November 2023, pp. 438–442, pubmed.ncbi.nlm.nih.gov/37781978/

highest mortality rate of any mental illness: N. Auger, B.J. Potter, U.V. Ukah et al., 'Anorexia nervosa and the long-term risk of mortality in women', *World Psychiatry*, vol. 20, no. 3, September 2021, pp. 448–449, ncbi. nlm.nih.gov/pmc/articles/PMC8429328/

autistic people generally do not respond as well to traditional eating disorder treatment models: S.L. Field, J.R.E. Fox, C.R.G. Jones et al., '"Work WITH us": a Delphi study about improving eating disorder treatment for autistic women with anorexia nervosa', *Journal of Eating Disorders*, vol. 11, no. 17, 2023, doi.org/10.1186/s40337-023-00740-z

Neurodivergent young adults are more likely than neurotypical teens: D. De Alwis, A. Agrawal, A.M. Reiersen et al., 'ADHD symptoms, autistic traits, and substance use and misuse in adult Australian twins', *Journal of Studies on Alcohol and Drugs*, vol. 75, no. 2, March 2014, pp. 211–221, ncbi.nlm.nih.gov/pmc/articles/PMC3965675/

more likely to have thoughts of suicide: P.I. Lin, W.T. Wu, E.K. Azasu et al., 'Pathway from attention-deficit/hyperactivity disorder to suicide/self-harm', *Psychiatry Research*, vol. 337, no. 115936, July 2024, pubmed. ncbi.nlm.nih.gov/38705042/; C.M. Conner, A. Ionadi and C.A. Mazefsky, 'Recent research points to a clear conclusion: autistic people are thinking about, and dying by, suicide at high rates', *The Pennsylvania Journal on Positive Approaches*, vol. 12, no. 3, November 2023, pp. 69–76.

Chapter 7: A neurosparkly adolescence

a smarter choice ecologically and economically: A. Stevenson-Hynes, 'Will switching to period underwear save you money?', Choice, 26 July 2022, choice.com.au/health-and-body/reproductive-health/womens-health/articles/will-switching-to-period-underwear-save-you-money

this increased need for sleep isn't laziness: Editors, 'Let teenagers sleep', *Scientific American*, 1 February 2023, scientificamerican.com/article/let-teenagers-sleep/

their first period between the ages of eight and eleven: O. Bellas and J. Shipman, '"It needs to be talked about earlier": some children get periods at 8, years before menstruation is taught at school', *The Conversation*, 9 February 2024, theconversation.com/it-needs-to-be-talked-about-earlier-some-children-get-periods-at-8-years-before-menstruation-is-taught-at-school-222887

Chapter 8: Adulting

much higher rates of unemployment: 'Autism and employment in Australia', Amaze, amaze.org.au/creating-change/research/employment/

those with ADHD also report challenges: Senate Standing Committees on Community Affairs, *Assessment and Support Services for People with ADHD*, 'Chapter 2 – The lived experience of ADHD', Parliament of Australia, 2023, aph.gov.au/Parliamentary_Business/Committees/Senate/Community_Affairs/ADHD/Report/Chapter_2_-_The_lived_experience_of_ADHD

the average young person will have up to seven different careers: S. Holder, 'Varied career prospects for Generation Z eases pressure of joining workforce, researcher says', ABC News, 25 July 2023, abc.net.au/news/2023-07-25/career-changes-bring-comfort-for-graduating-students/102638556

Chapter 9: Adult diagnosis

autism and ADHD tend to run in families: S.-L. Ma, L.H. Chen, C.-C. Lee et al., 'Genetic overlap between attention deficit/hyperactivity disorder and autism spectrum disorder in *SHANK2* gene', *Frontiers in Neuroscience*, vol. 15, no. 649588, 2021, ncbi.nlm.nih.gov/pmc/articles/PMC8111170/

at higher risk of sexual assault: V.O. Gotby, P. Lichtenstein, N. Långström et al., 'Childhood neurodevelopmental disorders and risk of coercive sexual victimization in childhood and adolescence – a population-based prospective twin study', *Journal of Child Psychology and Psychiatry*, vol. 59, no. 9, September 2018, pp. 957–965, pubmed.ncbi.nlm.nih.gov/29570782/

Index